Practical Public Health Nutrition

Roger Hughes and
Barrie M. Margetts

WILEY-BLACKWELL

A John W

This edition first published 2011

Blackwell Publishing Ltd was acquired by John Wiley & Sons in February 2007. Blackwell's publishing programme has been merged with Wiley's global Scientific, Technical, and Medical business to form Wiley-Blackwell.

Registered office
John Wiley & Sons Ltd, The Atrium, Southern Gate, Chichester, West Sussex, PO19 8SQ, United Kingdom

Editorial offices
9600 Garsington Road, Oxford, OX4 2DQ, United Kingdom
2121 State Avenue, Ames, Iowa 50014-8300, USA

For details of our global editorial offices, for customer services and for information about how to apply for permission to reuse the copyright material in this book please see our website at www.wiley.com/wiley-blackwell.

Wiley publishes its books in a variety of electronic formats: ePDF 9781444329216; ePub 9781444329223

Library of Congress Cataloging-in-Publication Data

Hughes, Roger, 1965–
    Practical public health nutrition / Roger Hughes and Barrie M. Margetts.
        p. ; cm.
    Includes bibliographical references and index.
    ISBN 978-1-4051-8360-4 (pbk. : alk. paper)
    1. Nutrition policy.   2. Public health.   3. Nutrition.   I. Margetts, Barrie M.   II. Title.
    [DNLM: 1. Nutrition Policy.   2. Public Health Practice.   3. Health Promotion.   4. Nutritional Physiological Phenomena.   QU 145 H894p 2011]
    TX359.H84 2011
    613.2–dc22

                                         2010022796

A catalogue record for this book is available from the British Library.

Set in 10/12.5 pt Times by Toppan Best-set Premedia Limited
Printed and bound in Singapore by Fabulous Printers Pte Ltd

1   2011

Contents

For our students and practitioner colleagues, past, present and future.
May they have as much positive impact on their populations as they have had on us.

Preface

Public health nutrition as a discipline and as a field of practice is of immense importance to human health and the societies in which we live. It is an area of work that is gathering momentum worldwide. The next few decades will be as challenging, if not more so, than those of the past. This book is a small but practical attempt to support the development of the public health nutrition workforce so that it has the capacity to address these challenges now and into the future. As an aspiring or current practitioner, we hope this book will confirm your current good practice or inform the process of practice improvement we consider so important if we are to have a genuine impact on public health.

The contents of this book have evolved over more than a decade of teaching nutrition and public health students about the practical applications of the principles, theories and processes used to develop population-based nutrition interventions. Over this period, we have come to recognise – albeit slowly – the importance of stepwise, purposive processes that integrate capacity building principles with conventional intervention planning, so that our work as practitioners produces sustainable outcomes (i.e. better nutrition and health) and sustainable activity (i.e. interventions continue beyond our involvement). As authors, our collective experience includes as much failure in practice as it does success. This experience has helped us identify what not to do, as much as it has identified what we must do to be more effective. So we don't pretend that we have all the answers or that this book in itself is enough to improve practice – that's ultimately up to you, the practitioner. But we hope that it helps in this process.

This book is called *Practical Public Health Nutrition* because it intentionally focuses on the principles and processes we believe are required to develop solutions to public health nutrition problems effectively. We introduce a new model to guide the systematic development, implementation and evaluation of interventions in practice. We acknowledge that it has been largely inspired by earlier work by many people and tempered by our own experiences in public health nutrition practice. We accept and emphasise that the practice of public health nutrition is still a work in progress. We hope that students and practitioners alike can use, develop and improve on the model and processes of practice that ultimately add to the effectiveness of public health nutrition effort and enhance public health. After all, that's what we are all about.

Roger Hughes and Barrie Margetts

Acknowledgements

This book has drawn on the scholarship and wisdom of many others and been tempered by our experiences as practitioners and teachers in this field of public health nutrition. We should, therefore, acknowledge those who have shaped our thinking and continue to question how best to address public health nutrition issues in practice. This includes our many colleagues and students who force us to continually reflect on what and how we practise and teach.

We would like to especially thank Christina Black who reviewed and commented on the whole manuscript, made important preparatory contributions to numerous chapters in this text, argued with us about the bi-cycle model and helped us make it more relevant to actual practice. Her fresh eyes and sharp intelligence, informed by experience as a public health nutrition practitioner, has been much appreciated.

Jenny Davies and Dr Nick Kennedy deserve mention for their collegial contributions to our discussions about this book which has indirectly influenced its content.

To the whole Blackwell team, thank you for your polite professionalism in making this book a reality.

To our respective partners and children, who support our work and careers in public health nutrition, continue to inspire us to do better and keep us grounded in what is important, may your lives continue to be interesting, happy and healthy.

Glossary

Action plans   Also known as strategic plans.

Best buys   Strategy initiatives with the greatest chance of achieving desired outcomes in a given context.

Capacity   The ability of a individual, organisation, community or population to achieve desired objectives (e.g. better health).

Capacity building   The process and practice of enhancing capacity.

Causal pathway   A relationship between exposures or determinants and outcomes that suggests causation.

Community development   A continuous striving to help develop the conditions for people to be inclusive, to share and care, so that they can live healthy, fulfilling lives.

Community engagement   The process of productively interacting with community members and relevant stakeholder groups.

Community organisation   The process of involving and mobilising a variety of agencies, institutions and groups in a community to work together to coordinate services and create programmes for the united purpose of improving the health of a community.

Competencies   The knowledge, skills and attitudes required to perform effectively in the workplace.

Core functions   Those functions that are regarded as absolutely necessary and without which would imply gaps in public health capacity.

Determinant analysis   Analysis of the factors that contribute to the expression of a health problem.

Downstream   Treatment-focused. Refers to the river of prevention analogy.

Economic evaluation   Economic evaluation involves identifying, measuring and valuing the inputs (costs) and outcomes (benefits) of intervention(s).

Effectiveness   The extent to which an intervention achieves the desired outcome in real-world settings/context.

Efficacy   The extent to which an intervention achieves the desired outcome in ideal settings/context.

Evaluability assessment   A process to assess if an intervention is ready to be evaluated.

Formative evaluation   Evaluation conducted to inform strategy development and evaluation planning.

Goal   The overarching change statement of the desired effect of the intervention.

Impact evaluation   Evaluation of intervention effects that relate to defined objectives and/or determinants.

Implementation failure   When interventions are not implemented as planned or inadequately implemented resulting in poor evaluation results.

Indicated prevention   Interventions targeted at high-risk individuals who are identified as having minimal but detectable signs or symptoms foreshadowing the specified health condition, or biological markers indicating a predisposition to it, but who do not currently fulfil diagnostic criteria.

Intelligence   Information from various sources and methods that help inform decision-making about intervention design.

Intervention management   The process and practice of developing, implementing, evaluating interventions, and sharing and applying the learning of this experience.

Intervention plan   A document that details the information required to effectively implement and intervention. An intervention blueprint.

Logic model   Usually a diagrammatic representation of the logic underpinning and intervention, which links identified determinants with intervention strategies and evaluation standards, making assumptions explicit about how the intervention is planned to bring about change.

Malnutrition   The abnormal physiological state associated with insufficient, excessive or imbalanced consumption of nutrients, characterised by an increased risk of morbidity and mortality. It refers to both under- and over-nutrition.

Mandates   Policy statements from organisations and institutions that sanction and prioritise action on nutrition issues.

Mixed-method evaluation   Evaluation that uses numerous methods to collect and analyse data to inform assessments of intervention effects.

Needs assessment   A formative evaluation process of assessing a populations need.

Objective   A statement of desired change in identified determinants of a nutrition problem. Usually written to be specific, measurable, achievable, realistic and time-limited.

Outcome evaluation   Asks the question: Has the intervention goal been achieved?

PEEST analysis   Situational analysis that considers the political, environmental, economic, social and technical dimensions of a health issue.

Primary prevention   Avoiding the onset of ill health and decreasing the number of new cases (the incidence).

Process evaluation   Asks the question: Was the intervention implemented as planned?

Professionalism   A state of mind and behaviour that reflects the mores and expectations of the professional community, often including personal behaviour and presentation, commitment to quality improvement and ethical practice.

Public health nutrition   The art and science of promoting population health status via sustainable improvements in the food and nutrition system. Based on public health principles, it is a set of comprehensive and collaborative activities, ecological in perspective and inter-sectoral in scope, including environmental, educational, economic, technical and legislative measures.

Reflective practice   A process in practice of reflecting on events or practices in order to understand and improve practice.

Reliability   Repeatability of a measure.

Reverse engineering   Deconstructing and backward analysis of strategies and interventions to critically assess the strategy/intervention logic.

Secondary prevention   Preventing the progression if ill health and reducing the rate of established cases in the community (the prevalence).

Stakeholder analysis   Identification, analysis and description of individuals, groups or organisations that have an interest in the issue being addressed.

Strategy portfolio   A mix of strategy options selected to achieve the best possible return on investment given context and available resources/opportunity.

SWOT analysis   Strengths, Weaknesses, Opportunity and Threats analysis.

Targeted prevention   Interventions targeted at individuals or a subgroup of the population whose risk of developing the health problem is significantly higher than average. The risk may be imminent or a lifetime risk.

Tertiary prevention   Stabilising or reducing the amount of disability and number of complications arising from an irreversible condition/disease.

Trial-and-error strategy development   Strategy development based on assumptions rather than by detailed analysis of the determinants of the nutrition issue.

Upstream   Prevention-focused. Referring to the river of prevention analogy.

Universal prevention   Interventions targeted at the general public or a whole population group that has not been identified on the basis of individual risk for the specified health problem. The intervention is desirable for everyone in that group.

Valorisation   The process of disseminating and exploiting the results of projects with a view to optimising their impact, transferring them, integrating them in a sustainable way and using them actively in systems and practices at local, regional, national and global levels.

Work package   A logical sequence or cluster of activities that relate to the development, implementation or evaluation of activities and strategies, reflecting the work required.

Part 1

Introduction and context

This introductory section comprises three chapters which provide the context for consideration of public health nutrition (PHN) as an area of practice. This context is important because it helps lays the foundation of a systematic and thorough approach to practice in public health nutrition discussed in later sections.

Chapter 1 provides a big picture overview of the immense challenges and complexity of PHN as a discipline. It also situates the practitioner in this context, arguing that effective practitioners can indeed make a difference to public health.

Chapter 2 defines PHN and describes its attributes as a practice area. Of equal importance, this chapter articulates what PHN is not, helping to situate it in the health system, with a focus on the protection, maintenance and promotion of health in different populations. This chapter has significant relevance to practitioners as it considers the core functions of the PHN practitioner and the associated competency needs.

Chapter 3 introduces and describes a bi-cycle framework for PHN practice which embeds capacity building with strategic and intelligence-based decision-making at the core of PHN practice. As a stepwise process, it is proposed as a model to assist the application of the rhetoric of health promotion in practice.

Chapter 1

The big picture: The context for a textbook on public health nutrition practice

Why develop a public health nutrition textbook?

This book has been written with the bold aim to help develop competent and effective public health nutrition (PHN) practitioners and to help existing practitioners work more effectively. In this context, the term practitioner refer to individuals or groups with an interest in, responsibility for or mandate to work in the interest of protecting and promoting public health through better nutrition. This can include local health workers, school teachers and hospital dietitians. In much of this book and for most readers it relates more to specialists, such as designated public health nutritionists – a role that is increasingly becoming established in many countries worldwide. It also refers to you, the reader, even if you currently do not have a formal qualification or professional status. We hope that this book, and the processes and principles it describes, will help develop and refine the competencies you require to be effective PHN practitioners. This is important because we contend that:

- there are currently many practitioners who aren't effective in a PHN context; and
- being effective is possible if we follow good practice.

Malnutrition is still the main game

It will come as no surprise that PHN practice is still dominated by considerations of malnutrition in its two-faced manifestations: under-nutrition and over-nutrition. At an international level there is little disagreement about the staggering burden of malnutrition in all its forms. It is now accepted that over a billion people across the world are under-nourished, with more now over-nourished and probably as many people with specific micronutrient deficiencies. Many of those who are under- or overweight are also micronutrient-deficient. Whereas in the past the burden of over-nutrition was highest in developed or rich countries, the burden is now spreading to and increasing in poor or developing countries. This trend is now referred to as the double burden of disease. In

Practical Public Health Nutrition, first edition. Roger Hughes and Barrie M. Margetts. Published 2011 by Blackwell Publishing Ltd. © 2011 Roger Hughes and Barrie M. Margetts.

some countries there is an additional burden associated with high rates of infectious diseases and/or HIV. There is a complex interplay between poverty, food and nutrition insecurity, malnutrition and infection that becomes a downward spiral, with infection adding to the metabolic demands for nutrition, while reducing the capacity to work and earn the money required to address the infection, which further reduces dietary intake. Thus a vicious cycle continues. These complex interactions spiral throughout the life-course, from infants to children, to young women having babies to babies. All this is exacerbated by basic and underlying causes, such as inequality, poverty, conflicts and natural disasters. Despite these enormous challenges, there have been improvements in some countries, but these have been largely offset by setbacks elsewhere.

Is food insecurity due to families being too large or wasting money on 'junk food', or are global food prices and the international controls on markets that make life difficult for the poorest in the least wealthy countries more to blame? Per capita food production has kept pace with the rise in population, but the biggest concern is that the rich world is consuming more than its fair share and producing more waste and greenhouse gases, while the poor are told to have fewer children so they can feed them (the same applies with consumption of fossil fuels). Food insecurity is a spectre hovering over humanity worldwide and it ebbs and flows with economic, political and environmental crises. This point was made clear in a recent FAO report on food insecurity in the world.[1] The nutrition challenges of today and into the future will continue to be essentially about inequality.

Innovative solutions are needed

The current approach to addressing global nutrition problems, articulated in many policies and resolutions at the international level, such as the Millennium Development Goals, the WHO resolution of diet, physical activity and health, etc., has moved to a model (some use the word paradigm) which relies on a therapeutic/technical approach. This involves giving supplements or fortifying staple foods as a key strategy to address the major micronutrient deficiencies of iron, vitamin A and iodine. In other words, the approach is to say, 'If we can't change the causes, we will treat the symptoms by giving what is missing'. Another competing paradigm argues that food is a fundamental human right and that, unless the basic causes of under-nutrition are addressed, until people have control over their lives and are consulted and become part of the solution rather than having solutions imposed on them, we will never fundamentally address health inequalities. So the challenges are enormous, but our work and role as practitioners may never be more important and needed.

Surely you don't mean these challenges can be found in rich countries like mine?

The challenges for public health nutritionists in developed or rich-economy countries are no less complicated that those of the developing world. What is consistent is the effect of socio-economic inequalities on malnutrition (the poor and uneducated also tend to be the most overweight) and the complex array of determinants that result in disease and disability. Under-nutrition still exists in vulnerable subpopulations and the enormous social burden of preventable disease attributable to over-nutrition makes the role of the public health nutritionist just as important in the developed world as in the developing world.

Level of influence

As a practitioner operating at a national or international level, the options for interventions or approaches to solving problems may be more linked to interventions that aim to improve nutrition by increasing the uptake of supplementation or supporting other attempts to diversify food intake at a national level. Or it may be that your role is to address national priorities, which in many countries are dominated by obesity. Many more of you will be working at a local level, where the policy, goals and objectives have already been set and your role may be to design, plan, implement and evaluate interventions that address the issues mandated in national action plans or priorities. Action by practitioners at all levels is required and important. The level at which you as a current or future practitioner operate will affect how much decision-making and influence you have over the approach to identifying problems and solutions, developing policy and delivering interventions. We argue, however, that at whatever level you operate, there is a practice model that you can work within which will help you be more effective in your practice context. This book outlines the steps in this practice model.

Practice informed by a public health approach

The values, attitudes and the conceptual approaches we apply to practice have a critical influence on our practice behaviours and overall effectiveness. A public health approach (described in more detail in later chapters) is traditionally defined by its focus on prevention rather than treatment, populations rather than individuals and interventions that address the determinants of health rather than the treatment of disease. It is an approach characterised by persistence, recognising that human health requires the right conditions and opportunities to flourish, and that we cannot afford to assume that these conditions will occur or persist without planned effort and attention. Such effort and attention are a key responsibility of the health workforce, policy-makers and community leaders.

First, work to understand the causes, by looking upstream

When we are taking a public health view it is important to step back from the problem and ask, 'Why did this problem arise?' In other words, we need to think about the underlying causes (determinants), such as 'Why did this child not have enough to eat or have diarrhoea? Was it because the household was food insecure or the family was poorly educated and had limited resources and access to education and health care?' Stepping back further the question is again 'Why is this so? Why is the family food insecure?' This is about having reliable and affordable access to nutritious food, as well as clean water and the means to cook. At the basic level the reason many households are food insecure is that the country is poor and has little capacity to generate jobs and provide services because they are dependent on low-yield cash crops as their major source of government revenue. UNICEF described this conceptual framework many years ago, which was updated in 2008 as part of the *Lancet* series reviewing the evidence around causes and solutions to under-nutrition in the world (see [2–6]).

Practitioners and politics

Turning the focus back to you as a practitioner, you may be asking if the problems are more to do with politics and decisions about fairness and equity, rights, trade and the capacity of countries to look after themselves. You may be wondering what you can possibly do to make a difference. The key point of the discussion in this chapter is to make sure that you consider the wider context in which the problem in front of you arose. If your responsibility is to reduce the prevalence of obesity, telling people to eat less fatty food may not be very effective if they cannot afford or have limited access to alternative, healthier foods. If your responsibility is to operate at a national or advisory level, again it may be helpful to reflect and think about the basic and underlying causes, and not rush in and 'treat' what may appear to be the obvious cause. In many countries, governments shy away from addressing these basic and underlying causes because they require them to take an active role – to introduce legislation or regulations that ensure people have enough to live on or that food manufacturers are regulated to optimise the healthfulness of their foods. Very often governments take the view that their role is to supply information and let the people decide, without addressing the real reasons why they are behaving as they do. It is well documented that only well-informed and edu-cated people read food labels and use that information to make decisions about what to buy. This may be one of the reasons for the widening gap! At the same time, the gov-ernment is often not enthusiastic to regulate, for example, which sugary/fatty snacks can be advertised on television at times when children, the target audience, are most likely to be watching. It may explain why governments are enthusiastic to urge people to be more active, but pay less attention to what industry is doing to the quality of the food supply.

The philosophy underpinning this book

There are two philosophical strands that underpin this book: first, that without well-trained and supported practitioners, even if we have excellent policies and statements of aims/goals and objectives, it is unlikely that effective interventions will be developed, delivered or evaluated; and second, that the approach to developing and addressing problems and the perspective one brings to the approach are critical.

Building capacity for effective public health nutrition action

In most reports on the global or national nutrition situation, few mention the workforce, its role or the skills and support the people doing the work need to be effective. To address this oversight, this book focuses on the practice of public health nutrition and the steps we must take in the development of strategic action and intervention, regardless of level or location in the system. PHN practice is evolving as the workforce of specialists worldwide develops. The UK, Australia and New Zealand have been among the countries that have begun to develop this workforce in recent years. In the US and Canada there is a long tradition of PHN jobs and roles. In all of these workforces, many of these roles are an extension of the treatment clinical model and do not really address a population, public health approach. Practice reorientation is needed if we are to be effective in addressing PHN issues. Be that as it may, we also argue that at whatever level and in whatever organisation you operate, the principles articulated in this book and captured in summary form in the bi-cycle model of PHN practice will help you make sense of where you are and what you need to do, help to explain why things are not working and help you build the evidence (intelligence) to inform your practice now and in the future. The bi-cycle has been developed, based on our own experience, successes, failures and frustrations in trying to develop, deliver and evaluate effective programmes aimed at improving health.

We end this chapter by suggesting 12 golden rules of PHN practice which we shall articulate through this book and which we hope will stay at the forefront of your mind throughout your career as public health nutritionists.

The 12 golden rules of public health nutrition practice

1. Know and engage thy community.
2. Seek first to understand and define the problem before acting.
3. Look upstream to determinants.
4. Recognise existing capacity and build, build, build.
5. Position activity within existing mandates.
6. Check what others have done and learnt, and use this intelligence.
7. Think first what can go wrong and manage the risks.
8. Pick the best options relative to context.
9. Use logic and plan, plan, plan.
10. Manage implementation so that your strategies are delivered as planned.
11. Evaluate, evaluate, evaluate.
12. Share what you learn, particularly your mistakes.

Chapter 2

Defining public health nutrition as a field of practice

Objective

By the end of this chapter you should be able to:

- Define public health nutrition as a field of practice distinct from other professional nutrition and broader public health practice, with reference to core work functions and competency requirements.

Introduction

There has been considerable debate over the last decade about what PHN is, how it is defined, what it involves and how it differs from well-established and known types of professional nutrition practice such as dietetics, and broader approaches to public health work evident in issues such as tobacco control, communicable diseases and injury prevention. This debate is important, particularly because PHN practice worldwide suffers from a lack of a public profile about the nature and utility of PHN work and the small number of formally named PHN positions.

PHN is not new, but the use of the title 'Public Health Nutritionist' to describe a professional and a recognition of the need for a specialist practitioner who deals with nutrition problems at a population level are increasingly becoming the focus of worldwide effort. The need for a recognised identity for public health nutrition as a specialised field of practice requiring a designated workforce is rooted in the realisation that the public health approach of prevention is likely to be a more cost-effective and sustainable course of action to control the worldwide chronic disease epidemic than traditional curative approaches.[7] This recognition has prompted efforts to build workforce capacity in public health nutrition.

Practical Public Health Nutrition, first edition. Roger Hughes and Barrie M. Margetts. Published 2011 by Blackwell Publishing Ltd. © 2011 Roger Hughes and Barrie M. Margetts.

Feature	Clinical dietetics	Community dietetics	Community nutrition	Public health nutrition
Setting	Hospitals	Community	Community	Community
Reach	Individuals	Individuals and small groups	Population sub-groups	Populations
Prevention	Secondary, tertiary, quaternary		Primary	
Paradigm	Illness		Wellness	
Key personnel	Dieticians and health workers		Many stakeholders, multidisciplinary and inter-sectoral	
Determinant of activity	Health worker referral		Community development, needs and policy directives	
Outcome timeframe	Short to medium		Medium to long	

Figure 2.1   Modes of nutrition practice
Source: Adapted from Hughes and Somerset.[8]

Modes of nutrition practice

A simple way of conceptualising PHN is to compare it with the various types of professional nutrition practice that are well known worldwide. In this approach, nutrition services can be considered as a continuum with overlap, delineated by setting, reach, type of prevention, care paradigm, key personnel, determinants of activity and outcome time-frame (see Figure 2.1).

   In reality, it is important to note that:

- any one practitioner may operate in each of these practice modes on any given day; and
- the methodology of community nutrition and public health nutrition is the same; population reach is the key difference.

   This book has been designed to help you work in the public health approach to practice and the following case study illustrates how different modes of practice produce different responses, require different resources and often produce different outcomes.

Case study: Comparison between different approaches to managing a communities problem with overweight and obesity

The traditional dietetic approach

Tony* is a dietician employed by the Southampton Community Health Centre. Data produced by the Area Health Epidemiology Unit have identified a recent increase in the prevalence of overweight and obesity in the area population and this finding is supported by an increasing rate of referral of overweight and obese clients to the health centre by general practitioners. Tony's initial response is to work with the other staff in the Community Health Centre to establish a multidisciplinary weight reduction clinic, linking with the local Division of General Practice. This results in a streamlined service providing services for an average of 60 individuals a week and occupying three days a week of his time. He notices that each individual needs an average of six visits over two to three months to stabilise their weight and sustain changes to related behaviours (the desired outcome), so there are ten outcomes per week. Realising that this method requires significant resources for the limited population reach, he reorganises the service into a group education format, increasing the client service rate to 120 per week for the same time investment and for twice as many outcomes per week (20). At this rate he will achieve about 1,000 outcomes each year.

The public health nutrition approach

Tess* is a public health nutritionist working for the Southampton Area Health Service and has decided to develop a PHN response to the spiralling rates of overweight and obesity in her community. The following account describes how each of the core functions listed in Table 2.4 applies to this scenario. Tess decides to act after analysing recently collected data from her epidemiology unit which show that the rates of overweight and obesity are increasing at an alarming rate, particularly among school children. Her first step is to consult key stakeholders in the community and form a representative taskforce to assist in planning a community-wide intervention to address the problem. At the same time as this taskforce is being established and commencing discussions, Tess lobbies her local public health unit to provide research support and some seed funding for the community taskforce to develop and implement its initial strategies. With the public health epidemiologist, Tess summarises the available public health data about overweight and obesity in a report that is used to inform the taskforce's deliberations and to communicate this information to the local health workforce. The taskforce then undertakes a determinant analysis (consultation, research and discussion to identify determinants of overweight and obesity in their community) assisted by Tess and staff from the public health unit. Their analysis shows that sedentary lifestyles and increasing reliance on takeaway food are the major direct determinants of increasing adiposity. Indirect determinants include a lack of community facilities for exercise, such as safe pathways, organised sports and affordable gym access. The increasing reliance on takeaway food is considered to be the result of time poverty among working parents, limited cooking skills, the saturation of the local community environment with fast-food advertising and the high number of fast-food outlets.

The taskforce develops a community strategy with Tess's assistance, who informs them about earlier interventions and their effectiveness and other possible options. This strategy forms the basis of a submission for funding from the state government to develop a community-wide obesity prevention strategy. Among other things, the strategy mix includes working with local government to:

- develop policies and invest in safe pathways;
- regulate fast-food outlets through town planning;
- introduce a train-the-teacher programme in district schools and health centres, so that teachers and health workers can implement a healthy meal preparation skills development programme for students, parents and other community members;
- develop a community sports organisation to coordinate community-wide physical activity for people of all ages, assisted by the Department of Sport and Recreation.

On receipt of government funding, Tess works with the taskforce and community stakeholders to implement the programme, making a concerted effort to keep stakeholders engaged in and informed about the project. The project team also develops community organisation systems and seeks funding to sustain the project after the government funding ends. On completion of the intervention funding, Tess works with stakeholders to evaluate the intervention and reports widely on its outcomes and lessons.

Comparison of approaches

The difference between these two approaches relates not only to the reach of the interventions, but also to the types of changes achieved, the determinants addressed and the competencies required to successfully implement them.

*The two scenarios in this case study are illustrative, and not based on real people or events.

Definitions of public health nutrition

Understanding what PHN practice involves, how it is performed and what it is trying to achieve is critical for effective action. Having statements that define PHN is important to provide a distinct professional identity, clear understanding and common professional vocabulary that describes and conceptualises PHN practice. Too inflexible a definition of PHN is not necessarily the best approach as a single definition may not fit the reality or needs of the workforce in different countries.

A number of approaches can be used to achieve a common understanding of PHN practice and avoid the constraint of a word-for-word definition. Such approaches include:

- exploration of existing definitions and definitional descriptors;
- exploration of the core functions (the required work) of PHN practice; and
- reflection on the competency requirements to perform this work.

Across the world various definitions of PHN have been developed over the last decade (Table 2.1).

From Table 2.1, it is clear that there are some attributes that are consistent among the definitions. The following definitional attributes (Table 2.2) have been identified in an international consensus development study,[14] further highlighting the consistently identified attributes of public health nutrition definitions.

The launch of New Nutrition Science[15] as a paradigm for nutrition sciences closely parallels these attributes of public health nutrition so it is not surprising that public health nutritionists do not consider the New Nutrition Science project as anything new, but see it as an important realisation of the complexity of nutrition as a field of research and practice, beyond the biological emphasis that has preoccupied the development of nutrition over the past century.

An emphasis on the *prevention* of food and nutrition problems

Public health nutrition as a discipline draws heavily on related fields, such as health promotion and public health. PHN practice is often similar to and draws on the principles and practice of health promotion – 'the process of enabling people to increase control over and to improve their health'.[16]

The defining features of a health promotion approach include actions that are:

- implemented across the whole population, not just those at risk of specific diseases;
- directed towards improving people's ability to control the factors that determine their health;
- part of a process involving a mix of strategies from a number of stakeholders which aim to improve health;
- focus on the prevention of disease and enhancement of health for all through tackling the social determinants of health.

Table 2.1   Definitions of public health nutrition from the literature

Source	Definition
Rogers & Schlossman (1997, USA)[9]	The term 'public nutrition' has been defined as a new field encompassing the range of factors known to influence nutrition in populations, including diet and health, social, cultural and behavioural factors; and the economic and political context. Like public health, public nutrition would focus on problem-solving in a real-world setting, making its definition an applied field of study whose success is measured in terms of effectiveness in improving nutrition situations.
Hughes & Somerset (1997, Australia)[8]	Public health nutrition is the art and science of promoting population health status via sustainable improvements in the food and nutrition system. Based on public health principles, it is a set of comprehensive and collaborative activities, ecological in perspective and inter-sectoral in scope, including environmental, educational, economic, technical and legislative measures.
Nutrition Society (Landman et al., 1998, United Kingdom[10]	PHN focuses on the promotion of good health through nutrition and the primary prevention of diet-related illness in the population. The emphasis is on the maintenance of wellness in the whole population.
Working group for the European Master's Programme for PHN (Yngve et al., 1999, European Union)[11]	PHN focuses on the promotion of good health through nutrition and physical activity and the prevention of related illness in the population.
Johnson (2001, (USA)[12]	PHN practice includes an array of services and activities to assure conditions in which people can achieve and maintain nutritional health, including surveillance and monitoring nutrition-related health status and risk factors, community or population based assessment, programme planning and evaluation, leadership in community/population interventions that collaborate across disciplines, programmes and agencies, and leadership in addressing the access and quality issues around direct nutrition services to populations.
Beaudry & Delisle (2005, Canada)[13]	Public['s] Nutrition applies the population health strategy to the resolution of nutrition problems, Its fundamental goal is to fulfil the human right to adequate food and nutrition. It is in the interest of the public, involves participation of the public and calls for partnership with relevant sectors beyond health.
World Public Health Nutrition Association (2007)	The promotion and maintenance of nutrition-related health and well-being of populations through the organised efforts and informed choices of society.

Table 2.2   Importance ratings for descriptors of how experts define the field of public health nutrition

	Very important	Important	Neutral	Not important	Very low importance
Population-based	23	1	0	0	0
Applies public health principles	17	4	3	0	0
Primary prevention	15	7	1	1	0
Focus on health promotion	14	9	0	1	0
Inter-sectoral action	13	6	3	1	0
Food and nutrition systems focus	12	10	0	1	0
Environmental	12	9	2	1	0
Political	12	9	2	1	0
Collaboration	11	7	4	1	0
Organised efforts	11	8	3	1	0
Wellness maintenance	10	10	3	1	0
Education	8	12	3	1	0
Economic	7	12	3	1	0
Leadership	7	10	3	3	0
Specifically includes physical activity within the definition	6	8	7	3	0
Behaviour change	6	13	4	1	0
Technical	5	8	10	1	0
Problem-oriented	5	10	5	3	1
Secondary prevention	4	9	7	3	1
Treatment	1	2	7	10	4

Source: From Hughes.[14]

The term 'prevention' is usually reserved for interventions that occur before the onset and diagnosis of a condition/disease is made.
  Prevention aims to:

• reduce the occurrence of new cases;
• decrease risk and/or increase protective factors that can be documented;
• delay the onset of illness;
• reduce the length of time that early symptoms continue; and/or
• halt the progression of severity.

In summary, prevention can be described as improving public health by adding years to life (i.e. increasing life expectancy, reducing premature death) and by adding life to years (i.e. improving the quality of life).

Conventionally, different levels of prevention are classified as:

Primary prevention	Avoid the onset of ill health and decrease in the number of new cases (*incidence*).
Secondary prevention	Prevent the progression of ill health and lower the rate of established cases in the community (*prevalence*).
Tertiary prevention	Stabilise or reduce the amount of disability and number of complications arising from an irreversible condition/disease.

The traditional classification system for prevention has been criticised as ambiguous and confusing. This system is suited to, and originally developed for, acute conditions with identifiable, uni-factorial causes, such as many infectious diseases. It is an inadequate model for complex, multi-factorial conditions such as obesity, Type 2 diabetes and cancers that have nutrition as a core determinant. With growing recognition that health is determined by multiple factors, an alternative classification system has emerged based on the level of intervention rather than the target outcome. Three types of interventions are outlined in the alternative prevention classification system shown in Table 2.3.

The core functions of the PHN workforce

PHN functions are defined as the work (processes, practices, services and programmes) carried out in order to promote health and well-being in populations through nutrition. PHN functions provide a description of the work required of practitioners and can be used as a benchmark against current work practices as a basis for workforce development.

There have been numerous and ongoing attempts worldwide to codify the core functions of the public health workforce in order to focus workforce practices and inform workforce development.[17,18]

Whilst it is logical to assume that the core functions for public health would also represent the core functions of PHN, there is widespread agreement that PHN is a specialty within public health requiring individual attention. Recent research from the European Union, based on earlier, worldwide workforce development research,[19,20] determined consensus on ten core functions for PHN (Table 2.4).

These core functions can be classified into three overarching function categories for PHN practice:

1 research and analysis;
2 building capacity; and
3 intervention management.

Table 2.3 Alternative prevention classification system

Category	Description	Examples for diabetes prevention
Universal	Interventions targeted at the general public or a whole population group that has not been identified on the basis of individual risk for the specified health problem. The intervention is desirable for everyone in that group.	Mass media programmes to promote fruit and vegetable consumption. Food advertising legislation against high fat, salt, sugar (HFSS) foods.
Selective	Interventions targeted at individuals or a subgroup of the population whose risk of developing the health problem is significantly higher than average. The risk may be imminent or it may be a lifetime risk. Risk groups may be identified on the basis of biological, psychological or social risk factors that are known to be associated with specific health problems.	Nutrition education for families with children identified as obese. Adoption of a healthy canteen policy in a workplace dominated by middle-aged office workers.
Indicated	Interventions targeted at high-risk individuals who are identified as having minimal but detectable signs or symptoms foreshadowing the specified health condition, or biological markers indicating predisposition to it, but who do not currently fulfil diagnostic criteria. These interventions can be applied to asymptomatic individuals with markers as well as to symptomatic individuals whose symptoms are insufficiently severe to warrant a diagnosis of a disorder.	Dietary prescriptions for people with identified glucose-resistance. Industry product modification (reduced sugar/fat/portion size) for high-risk individuals.

These core functions serve as a framework for PHN practice and are underpinned by the following assumptions:

- Public health nutrition functions are defined as those activities (processes, practices, services and programmes) undertaken by the workforce in order to promote optimal nutrition, health and well-being in populations.
- Core PHN functions are those functions that are regarded as absolutely necessary and without which would imply gaps in public health capacity.

Table 2.4 Ten core functions for public health nutrition practice

	Core public health nutrition function
Research & analysis	1 Monitor, assess and communicate population nutritional health needs and issues. 2 Develop and communicate intelligence* about determinants of nutrition problems, policy impacts, intervention effectiveness and prioritisation through research and evaluation.
Build Capacity	3 Develop the various tiers of the PHN workforce and its collaborators through education, disseminating intelligence* and ensuring organisational support. 4 Build community capacity and social capital to engage in, identify and build solutions to nutrition problems and issues. 5 Build organisational capacity and systems to facilitate and coordinate effective public health nutrition action.
Intervention management	6 Plan, develop, implement and evaluate interventions that address the determinants of priority public health nutrition issues and problems and promote equity. 7 Enhance and sustain population knowledge and awareness of healthful eating so that dietary choices are informed choices. 8 Advocate for food and nutrition-related policy and government support to protect and promote health. 9 Promote, develop and support healthy growth and development throughout all life-stages. 10 Promote equitable access to safe and healthy food so that healthy choices are easy choices.

*Intelligence refers to information and knowledge from various sources that is used to inform decisions relating to problem resolution in public health nutrition practice.
Source: From Hughes.[21]

- The relative importance of functions may vary according to the jurisdiction or workforce level.
- Core functions are interrelated and complementary.
- Core functions articulate the work required to effectively address PHN problems or issues, and consequently provide a framework for identifying and conceptualising workforce development needs.
- Current PHN work practices do not accurately align with these core functions.[23]

These core functions are aspirational and outline the practices required for effective PHN action that can be used to improve practice.

Competencies for PHN practice

Competencies are the knowledge, skills and attitudes required to work effectively. Competency standards (a codified statement of required competencies) may guide practitioners in defining the knowledge, skills and experience required to undertake PHN practice.

Over the past decade work has been undertaken to develop consensus on the elements of competency required by the PHN workforce. In summary, the competencies include a number of specific elements and performance criteria under the broad competency groupings of:

- foundation and theoretical knowledge and skills;
- analysis;
- public health service;
- socio-cultural and political context;
- management and leadership; and
- professionalism and communication.

The PHN competencies provide a structure for:

- *Curriculum design and evaluation* – by ensuring competency development through teaching and learning to correspond with agreed competency needs.
- *Credentialing* – by providing standards that can be used as benchmarks for practitioner recognition or registration.
- *Performance review* – by providing standards which enable employers and practitioners to review practises and development needs.
- *Recruitment* – by providing a framework for articulating the competency and qualification expectations in position descriptions (duty statements, selection criteria).
- *Career planning* – by providing direction for individual practitioners considerations about further development needs.

Professionalism and PHN practice

Many of the competency expectations required of public health nutritionists reflect professionalism.

Professionalism entails practitioners drawing on relevant knowledge and applying professional responsibilities and ethical principles to their practice. Professionalism is associated with respectful self-presentation, a caring attitude, interpersonal competence and commitment to lifelong learning. There are three key dimensions in professionalism:[22]

- being knowledgeable;
- being empathetic;
- being reflective.

The *knowing* dimension relates to the concept of lifelong learning and the acquisition and appropriate application of knowledge. This dimension includes a commitment to *evidence-based practice* through the *attainment of intelligence* and information from a range of sources which are used to make informed decisions and interventions.

Development of competencies for practice and *continued professional/competency development* is included in the knowledge dimension of professionalism. Drawing on prior knowledge, using various learning methods and incorporating social and cultural knowledge domains develop expertise and innovation and increase knowledge of the broader determinants of health and context of practice.

The *empathetic* dimension is concerned with the moral-ethical sensitivity of health practice and the universal nature of human problems. This dimension includes a commitment to *ethical and moral practice*, the promotion of citizenship and an *obligation to human rights*. Health is a basic human right and there is a need to ensure that professional practice aims to reduce inequalities in health. Empathetic exchange between the professional and community/population must be established for social transformation and *capacity building* to occur, as well as for intervention success and improved health outcomes.

The *reflective* dimension involves *reflecting on action* whereby practitioners step back from practice and takes a broad view to understand *what activities have worked or failed and why*. Such reflective practice enables practitioner to link theory and practice by understanding how theory can assist practice and how practical experience can contribute to a wider theoretical understanding. Reflective practice ensures that attention is paid to both objective and subjective learning experiences which make an important contribution to the intelligence of practice.

Key points

- Public health nutrition is an evolving area of practice. As a consequence it is important to define clearly and conceptualise public health nutrition as a discipline in practice.
- PHN practice is primarily about problem-solving – developing interventions in the population that address the socio-cultural, economic, environmental and individual determinants of suboptimal nutrition.
- PHN practice can best be defined by the nature of the work or core functions and by an understanding of the competencies required to perform this work

Chapter 3

A framework for public health nutrition practice

Objectives

By the end of this chapter you should be able to:

- Describe they key steps in the PHN intervention practice bi-cycle.
- Explain the importance of integrating capacity building with intervention planning processes.

Introduction

As practice in public health nutrition implies doing something beyond analysis or contemplation about nutrition problems, one of the initial challenges is working out what to do first, when, how and with whom. Experience with working with colleagues who are new to PHN practice (usually clinically experienced dietitians who have made a career path change into PHN or relatively new graduates) has reinforced the need to develop a step-by-step guide to developing population-based interventions. In this context, practice is defined as all the work you do to effectively develop, implement and evaluate interventions that solve population-based nutrition problems. The essence of practice is developing solutions to established problems in communities of different sizes, structures and contexts. This means that practice is dynamic, contextual and complicated. This chapter describes a stepwise framework for practice that is systematic and process-driven, to help bring order to this complexity.

A socio-ecological approach to practice

The socio-ecological approach is often referred to as an *upstream approach* because it operates from a premise that health opportunities are not distributed randomly within populations, but instead the determinants of public health are embedded in the social, cultural, economic, environmental and other circumstances in which people live (collectively, the 'ecology'). It focuses on addressing determinants of public health and the outcomes of interventions are measured in terms of change to determinants (e.g. better education, social cohesiveness, cooking skills, etc.), as well as changes in health outcomes (e.g. fewer obesity-related deaths). This approach encourages practitioners to look *upstream* at determinants as a basis for intervention, change and evaluation, often with the underlying causative logic that if we change what causes the problem, the impacts of the problem will decrease or disappear. This is the basis of *logic modelling*, which is an intervention designing device which will be covered in later chapters. This approach closely parallels the major ideological thrust underpinning the New Nutrition Science project.[15]

Upstream vs. downstream: the river of prevention analogy

Consider a scenario where you approach a river and notice lots of people in the water struggling to stay afloat and at great risk of drowning. You have a number of options for intervening to address this problem (that people are drowning).

A *downstream* approach is to jump into the river and use your advanced surf lifesaving skills honed on the beach in Australia, retrieve each person one-by-one and give mouth-to-mouth resuscitation. After three hours of intense effort you have managed to save ten people, but 35 have drowned because you didn't have the capacity to save them all.

An *upstream* approach would be to run upstream and fence off the river at the point where people fall in so that they are no longer at risk of drowning. This saves almost everyone from drowning because it practically eliminates their exposure to the river and the risk of drowning. It does however take time and does nothing to save those already in the water.

Both approaches have their applications and limitations. Upstream approaches, however, are arguably more direct and effective forms of prevention.

The PHN practice cycle

PHN practice borrows heavily from the related disciplines of health promotion, public health and dietetics, and has adopted many of the practice cycles that have evolved in these disciplines. Because PHN practice is directed towards actions based on the personal, cultural, social, political and environmental determinants of health, the interaction and varying mix of determinants in different communities will vary, making PHN practice sensitive to context and circumstances. Because of the many interrelated factors influencing nutrition and health, it is necessary to develop a strategic and contextual approach to plan and develop programmes to protect and promote the health of the people.

Cyclical processes for intervention management

There have been numerous cyclical conceptualisations of health promotion practice which have been embraced by public health nutrition.[23] Cyclical processes for interven-

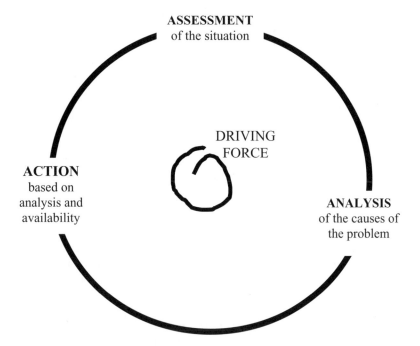

Figure 3.1   The Triple A cycle
Source: Adapted from www.unsystem.org/scn/archives/tanzania/ch05.htm.

tion management and practice have been used for many years and vary to their degree of segmentation in the stepwise cycle. The *Triple A cycle*[24] (Figure 3.1) includes three main steps of Analysis, Action and Assessment and was developed in Africa in the 1980s to assist with interventions dealing with malnutrition.

Figure 3.2 represents the stepwise PHN cycle borrowed from health promotion to describe the nature of PHN practice. This model replicates the basic cycle of needs assessment, planning, implementation and evaluation used in earlier health promotion planning models. As a model for informing PHN practice, it is limited by its simplicity and tells us little about the 'how to' questions which are of such relevance to practitioners.

Recognising the importance of capacity building as a discrete strategy and as an approach to practice

The most basic definition of capacity is the ability of a community or intervention team to achieve stated objectives. Capacity building is a core function of the PHN workforce and is critical to effective practice.[25] The importance of capacity building as a determinant of intervention success is often overlooked.

Capacity building has been referred to as the invisible work of health promotion because it is often done behind the scenes, rather than as a specific and overt strategy.

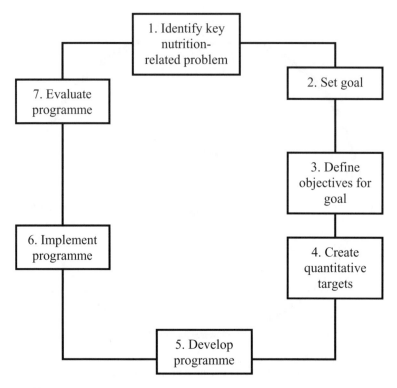

Figure 3.2 The public health nutrition cycle
Source: Adapted from Margetts.[23]

The invisibility of capacity building has been described as being the result of a failure of practitioners and resource allocators to recognise the importance and potential of capacity building activities to be a cost-efficient and value-adding approach to practice.[26]

A failure to build capacity around an intervention (e.g. by engaging the community, accessing and mobilising resources, building teams, etc.) will result in disappointing intervention implementation (implementation failure) and a resulting lack of health gain. It has been argued that capacity building strategies and evaluation in practice should be made visible, communicated, debated and recognised by practitioners and resource allocators as important and legitimate strategies.[25] The practice framework shown in Figure 3.3 overlays capacity building processes and strategy with intervention planning processes to form an integrated system for practice.

This model attempts to integrate capacity building with project planning cycles, making capacity building explicitly a core component of PHN intervention management. While this model integrates capacity building with intervention management processes to represent good practice more satisfactorily, it is limited by the stationary nature of the cycle (although in practice it may feel like we are going round in circles and getting

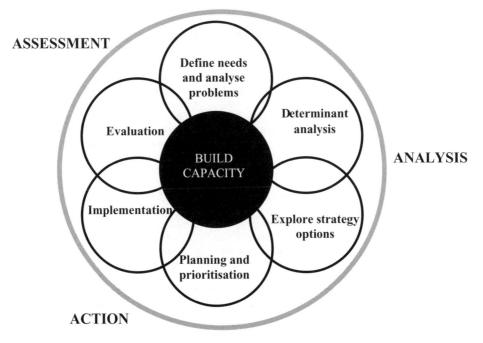

Figure 3.3   Public health nutrition intervention management practice cycle
Source: From Baillie et al.[25]

nowhere). This is not the intention of cyclical processes, which assume that the cyclical process moves forward our effectiveness in dealing with PHN issues. Each stage of the planning framework is briefly described and will form the cycle of practice that comprises the basis for the rest of this course.

Why make things more complicated and introduce a new framework?

PHN practice is dynamic and evolving. As authors of earlier versions of PHN practice models described earlier, we acknowledge that each model wasn't a perfect fit (if there is such a thing). The main limitations (frustrations) with these models are that:

- They are too simplistic, although they appear to be getting more detailed with each iteration, and don't adequately deconstruct practice in a way that can inform responses to the 'where do I start, how and with whom?' questions.
- They do not reflect progress in practice – moving forward rather than going round in circles.
- They do not adequately integrate capacity building strategies with project planning in a step-by-step sequence.

Table 3.1 Capacity prerequisites and capacity gain at each stage of the public health nutrition intervention management cycle

Stage		Suggested capacity prerequisites	Capacity gain examples
ASESSMENT	Define needs and analyse problems	Need and problem analysis requires access to information derived from research, community and stakeholder consultation and appropriate analytical expertise.	The act of consultation, collation of information and analysis has independent capacity building effects. Stakeholders and communities can be empowered through genuine consultation and community priorities can be identified.
ANALYSIS	Determinant analysis	Isolation and description of the social, economic, environmental and physical determinants (causative and protective factors) of public health problems require similar prerequisites as above.	Dissemination of determinant analysis results to stakeholders and communities can facilitate shared understanding and decision-making regarding priorities and strategy options.
ANALYSIS	Explore strategy options	Access to intervention research findings (evidence there the strategies have worked before) and practice wisdom.* Consultation and involvement of the community and stakeholders about potential solutions.	Shared decision-making about strategy options can empower stakeholders and encourage later target group engagement in interventions.
ACTION	Planning	Planning expertise, such as familiarity with logic modelling, project management and leadership.	Participation of stakeholders in planning can be empowering (as in shared decision-making). Well-developed plans provide a structural platform for effective intervention implementation.
ACTION	Implement the strategy portfolio	Resources, commitment and engagement by stakeholders.	Implementation (the 'doing' phase) can consolidate partnerships and encourage ongoing consultation and community development.
ASESSMENT	Evaluation	Evaluation skills, access to data, target group consultation and detailed understanding of the intervention logic and context. Evaluation should answer the question of whether the intervention has achieved its goals and objectives and sustained outcomes and effects.	Evaluation and reflection on strategies and decision-making can enhance shared understanding, build intelligence and share learning. The experience of implementation as measured in process evaluation can support sustainable gains in community competence in problem-solving.

*Practice wisdom refers to the knowledge and insights gained from experience in practice, based on observation, previous anecdotal or empirical evaluation and reflective practice.
Source: From Baillie et al.[25]

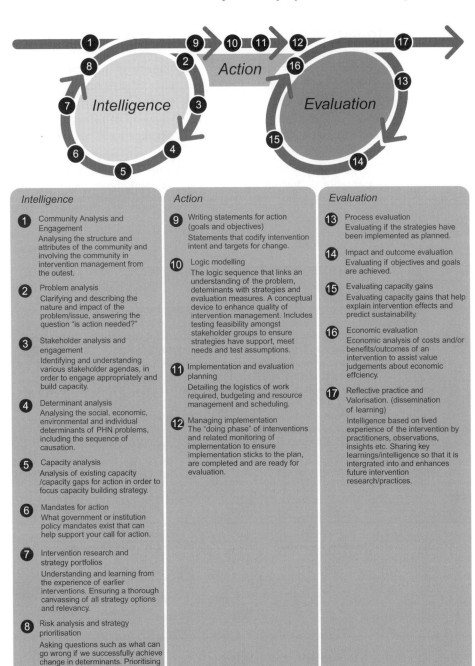

Figure 3.4   The public health nutrition practice bi-cycle

A bi-cyclic framework for public health nutrition practice

Building on these earlier cyclical models, the following framework forms the stepwise basis for the 17 steps that are involved in PHN intervention management (Figure 3.4). While essentially a twist on the cyclical models and an adaptation of the Triple A cycle, it conceptually recognises the progressive and cumulative nature of PHN practice (i.e. moving forward) and integrates capacity building into a planning → implementation → evaluation sequence.

This practice framework forms the basis for the following chapters and emphasises the process, tools and rationale for practice approaches in public health nutrition. It is intentionally pedantic in the way that it has deconstructed earlier models into what may seem to be overly numerous discrete steps.

Key points

- PHN practice needs to be dynamic, responsive and contextual to the setting, situation and available resources.
- PHN practice models have been evolving and are getting more complex. This complexity underscores the importance of detailed analysis of intelligence, strategic development of interventions (action) and attention and rigour in evaluation.
- Capacity building is central to PHN practice effectiveness, as a discrete strategy and as an approach to practice. It needs to be included and integrated into intervention management processes.
- The bi-cyclic framework for practice has a detailed, integrated and progressive emphasis and provides a basis for accumulative PHN practice.

Part 2

Intelligence

This section has eight chapters which describe the first steps in the PHN practice cycle. The intelligence phase of PHN practice, represented by the first loop in the bi-cycle, forces us to *understand before acting*. The risk of not understanding before acting is that our effort and other resources are applied ineffectively and our interventions fail. Understanding before acting means careful and detailed analysis of the community, its capacity for action, the problems it is facing and what determinants have a causal relationship with the problem, the rationale being that unless we understand what upstream factors (determinants) need to be changed, it is difficult to develop strategies that will lead to a change in the downstream issues being addressed.

Chapter 4

Step 1: Community engagement and analysis

Objectives

By the end of this chapter you should be able to:

1. Explain the importance of community and stakeholder engagement at the outset of intervention management.
2. Describe the various constructs and concepts underpinning community development.
3. Identify key dilemmas and influences of community development.
4. Demonstrate how community development and empowerment builds capacity.
5. Describe strategies for community engagement in the context of public health nutrition intervention management.
6. Conduct a community analysis.

Practical Public Health Nutrition, first edition. Roger Hughes and Barrie M. Margetts. Published 2011 by Blackwell Publishing Ltd. © 2011 Roger Hughes and Barrie M. Margetts.

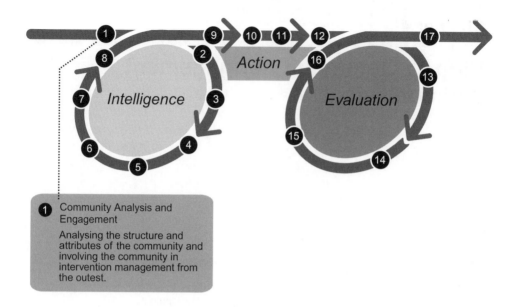

① Community Analysis and
Engagement

Analysing the structure and
attributes of the community and
involving the community in
intervention management from
the outest.

Introduction

One of the defining features of PHN practice is its focus on populations or communities rather than individuals. Populations are complex and dynamic, so it is important not only to 'know thy community' but also to engage the community in our approach to work – in other words, making sure the 'public' is central to PHN practice. This engagement can take many forms and is rooted in the belief that communities already have significant internal capacity to rise to challenges, when required. It may include consultation, observation and analysis to an extent that it enhances understanding about the community context. Community engagement not only serves to provide intelligence to inform intervention design, but also acts as a strategy that empowers communities, builds capacity and enhances the sustainability of PHN actions.

What is a community?

Populations, the focus of PHN practice, are made up of communities. A community is generally defined by its homogeneous unity. The most commonly cited factors for defining community or population include:

- *Geographical proximity* – assumes that people living in the same area have the same neighbourhood concerns.
- *Cultural similarity* – assumes common cultural traditions transcend geographical barriers and unite disparate groups of people.
- *Social stratification* based on common interests or characteristics – members often share support networks, knowledge and resources that transcend geographical and other boundaries.[27]

It is important to note that people may belong to several communities within a population, have varying degrees of commitment and the significance of a community may differ across life-stages. Within a community, people interact with each other and their ecology (social, physical, policy environments). This interaction is a significant determinant of the community's health status.

Why community engagement?

PHN practice enables people to increase control over and improve their nutrition-related health. Effective PHN practice involves engaging the community or population in the first stages of the practice bi-cycle, recognising the value of community-based resources, such as knowledge, local leadership and other determinants of capacity. Successful preventative health interventions are greatly dependent on the participation and support of the community in which they are developed and implemented.

Effective and sustainable outcomes are unlikely if health professionals plan interventions without consulting stakeholder groups or believe (and act as if) they are the experts and know what is best for the community. Effective PHN practitioners are those that act as *catalysts for community action* and who empower others to develop intelligent strategies to deal with identified determinants of nutrition-related health problems. In simple terms, community engagement in PHN practice involves *ongoing* consultation and support to develop the community's confidence, skills and resources to identify, prioritise, organise and collectively solve its nutrition-related health problems. The ability of a community to take action and achieve its objectives (such as dealing with a health issue) is often referred to as community capacity.[28]

It should be noted that community engagement and development are not structured or formulaic processes but need to be adapted and informed by the community itself in the context of individual communities.[29] The following poem adapted from one by Chabot (1976) reflects the community engagement and development approach to building community capacity in PHN practice.

> Go to the people
> Live among them
> Talk with them
> Start with what they know
> Build on what they have
> Identify and support leaders
> When their task is accomplished
> Their work is done
> The people all remark
> We have done it ourselves
> … And the PHN can move onto other issues

Practice note

Who best represents a community?
One of the challenges of community engagement is identifying who in the community best represents the community. Individuals with the time, energy and motivation to participate in PHN interventions may not represent or understand the issues as experienced by the most needy in the community. Beware the dominant minority. Explore a mix of strategies to identify and engage those most affected by the issue you are dealing with.

Community development constructs

There are several constructs and methods underpinning community development that must be explored to assist in the consideration of strategies and planning for community engagement to enhance PHN capacity. The key community development constructs of participation, empowerment, equity and community organisation and action are outlined in Table 4.1.

Table 4.1   Community development constructs

Construct	Description
People's participation	The term 'participation' is generally used to refer to processes of communication and joint action between communities and health development workers. The purpose of such participatory processes is usually the planning and implementation of community development strategies and health services which are responsive to community-determined health needs and which are sensitive to the political, social and economic realities of the context in question.[30] Consultation (rather than participation) occurs when decisions have already been made and there is little likelihood of change being made, although people are still asked to comment on the plan. Consultation is a poor substitute for true participation in the planning process.[31]
Empowerment	Empowerment as a construct emphasises individual and collective actions focused on capacity building and shifts in power and control over decisions and resources. It is the means by which people experience more control over decisions that influence their health and lives. More specifically defined as shifts towards greater equality in the social relations of power (who has resources, authority, legitimation or influence).[32] It is only by being able to organise and mobilise oneself that individuals, groups and communities will achieve the social and political changes necessary to redress their powerlessness and take control over their lives.[33] Key characteristics of empowerment: • it applies to the individual and the collective/community; • it addresses the issue of power and control over resources and the direction of one's own life; • it addresses issues of capacity and confidence building of both individuals and communities; and • it identifies active participation as a necessary but insufficient contribution.
Equity	Equity in health refers to acknowledging health inequalities and prioritising activities with those who stand to benefit the most and whose needs are greatest. Addressing inequalities involves examining the provision, quality, accessibility and availability of services and conditions required for health.[31]
Community organisation and collective action	Community organisation is the process of involving and mobilising a variety of agencies, institutions and groups in a community to work together to coordinate services and create programmes for the united purpose of improving the health of a community.[29] This process requires the development of effective partnerships and alliances between agencies from a wider spectrum than just the health sector. Collective action occurs when people act jointly to bring about changes in their circumstances that they identify need to be changed. Collective action is the visible evidence that community development is successful.[31]

Community development – a process or an outcome?

Community development has been commonly viewed in the literature as both a process and an outcome. As an outcome, community development or empowerment as an interplay between individual and community change has a long time-frame, typically 5–10 years or longer. At the individual level, people may experience a more immediate psychological empowerment.

Community development or empowerment is most consistently viewed in the literature as a process in the form of a dynamic continuum, involving personal empowerment, the development of small, mutual groups, community organisations, partnership, and social and political action. The potential of community development and empowerment is gradually maximised as people progress from individual to collective action along this continuum.[34]

Community development dilemmas and influences

Evidence suggests that social support and community involvement bring about health-enhancing benefits and can produce sustainable changes to the *upstream* determinants of health. However, there are many challenges and dilemmas involved in community development work. Adhering to the fundamental principles of community development; equality, participation, preventive action, commitment to partnerships and collective action and empowerment of individuals and communities can be a lengthy process, with a lack of tangible results or changes in health outcomes.

There are four identified dilemmas or influences that have an impact on community development practice:

1 *Funding* – funding is frequently provided on a short-term basis and may have pre-identified areas of focus determined by the funding agency. Short-term funding can increase the chance of problems with planning and/or evaluation due to time and resource limitations.

2 *Accountability* – dual accountability commonly exists in community development practice, with accountability to (a) funding agency/employer and (b) the community. Issues can emerge if there are conflicting priorities or differing responses to an issue. As a result, the practitioner can spend considerable time acting as a mediator.

3 *Acceptability* – community development practice may not always be accepted or condoned by employers or organisational management because of the time and resource requirements without the guarantee of health-related results. Acceptability of the practitioner by the community can also be an initial issue, particularly if the community has seen a high turnover of service providers or the practitioner is not an identified community member. There is a need to build trust, share knowledge and experiences and develop relationships before progress can begin.

4 *Professional attitude* – taking the attitude that you are an expert in the field and know what is best for the community can cause issues in community development practice. The role of the practitioner in community development practice is to be a catalyst and a facilitator, rather than an expert. Such practice involves developing egalitarian relationships and two-way knowledge sharing. For health professionals

whose identity is tied to their expert role, this shift in professional practice may be difficult.[27]

Building community capital (and capacity)

A healthy community is one that has high levels of social, ecological, human and economic 'capital', the combination of which may be thought of as 'community capital'.[33]

The term 'capital' indicates wealth and comes from the recognition that health is a form of wealth, and while human health is a key element of human capital, for a community to be healthy all four forms of capital need to increase together. A review by the World Bank showed that 60% of the world's wealth was found in human and social capital, indicating the importance of focusing on human and social development and that economic activity is a means to achieve this development.

These four types of capital, identified by Hancock,[33] are relevant to community engagement and capacity building in PHN practice and reinforce the importance in prioritising effort towards community development to produce social and human capital gain.

When analysing resource requirements for public health effort and interventions, it can be easy to focus on insufficient money or staff capacity or lack of equipment to complete the tasks. Whilst this is important and in most cases probably true to an extent, it is important not to focus purely on the lack of funding available to do things. A prioritisation of effort to community capacity building and emphasising the value of investing in social and human capital gain, ahead of the use of public health resources for direct or professional-lead interventions, is warranted.

The basic principle is: use what you already have before asking for external funding.

Case study: Community capacity outcomes from community gardens

Developing community gardens as a strategy to increase the availability of fruit and vegetables has additional benefits in terms of community development and community capacity building. Evidence suggests that community gardens facilitate *improved social networks* and *organisational capacity of the community*. Community gardens in lower socio-economic areas have provide a symbolic focus which *increases neighbourhood pride* and the *aesthetic maintenance of neighbourhoods*.

Community gardens have been shown to contribute to all four forms of community capital:

- *Social capital* – Development and management of community gardens require members to build cohesive social networks that often cross ethno-racial divides and lead to collective action to address broader community concerns.
- *Human capital* – Improved knowledge and skills in gardening, other cultures, cooking and nutrition, the environment and organic gardening, and intergenerational learning.
- *Ecological capital* – neighbourhood oasis of green space, flowers, insects and birds, along with adoption of organic farming practices and reduced waste production from composting.
- *Economic capital* – gardens can help reduce the cost of living by providing cheaper food sources, increasing disposable income and contributing to the local food bank or commercial production.

Source: From Hancock[33] and Armstorng.[34]

Table 4.2 Four forms of capital that contribute to community capital

Type of capital	Description	Contribution to global wealth
Social capital	The glue that holds communities together. It has an informal aspect related to social networks and a more formal aspect related to social development programmes. High levels of social capital are rooted in informal social networks that have been termed 'social cohesion' and 'civic-ness' and in participation in society, including the governance processes through which decisions are made. More informal forms of social capital can result from society's investment in social development ensuring equitable access to basic determinants such as peace, safety, food, shelter, education, income and employment.	60% social and human capital
Human capital	Healthy, well-educated, skilled, innovative and creative people engage in their communities and participate in governance. The end point: the central purpose of human-centred development.	
Natural capital	High environmental quality, healthy ecosystems, sustainable resources and the conservation of habitat, wildlife and biodiversity. Constitutes the bedrock of our society.	20%
Economic capital	The means by which we can attain many of our human and social goals (clean water, sanitation, food, housing, etc.). Economic capital can and should create healthy jobs and its equitable distribution ensures that people's basic needs are met. However, the means of increasing economic capital must not threaten our human capital, environmental or social capital on which we depend for our health and well-being.	20%

Source: Adapted from Hancock.[33]

Building capacity via 'bottom-up' practice

As a practitioner or student in public health or related areas you may have experience and knowledge in programme planning or intervention management. However, the constructs of community development and capacity building can present challenges for health professionals because they necessarily involve health practitioners relinquishing

Table 4.3   Key differences between top-down and bottom-up approaches

	Top-down	Bottom-up
Root/cause of problem	Individual responsibility	Empowerment
Approach	Weakness/deficit Solves problem	Strength/capacity Improves competence
Definition of problem	Determined by outside agent: government agency	By community
Primary vehicles for health promotion and change	Education, lifestyle change, improved services	Building community control, resources and capabilities towards social, economic and political change
Role of outside agents	Service delivery Resource allocation	Respond to needs of community
Primary decision-makers	Agency representatives, business leaders, 'appointed community leaders'	Indigenous/local community-appointed leaders
Community-controlled resources	Low	High
Community ownership	Low	High
Evaluation	Quantifiable outcomes and targets	Pluralistic methods documenting changes of importance to community

Source: Adapted from Lavarack and Labonte.[35]

control and working towards role obsolescence. Essentially, our work in public health is largely complete if we have managed to build, empower and organise communities to develop and implement solutions in a sustainable way, so that the community is no longer reliant on health practitioners. Capacity building as a feature of PHN practice should aim to make our role redundant. Whilst this ambition is nice in principle, the reality is that communities may not have the capacity to change factors beyond community control, such as world trade and tariff protection and other competing groups that drive government policy that facilitate/inhibit effective programme delivery.

Lavarack and Labonte[35] have argued that two, seemingly different discourses in health promotion have emerged in programme planning: *top-down* and *bottom-up*. The key differences between these two approaches are shown in Table 4.3.

Community engagement as a strategy in a capacity building approach can thus be described as a *bottom-up* approach, informed and owned by the community. Lavarack and Labonte concede, however, that top-down programmes follow a predetermined

Table 4.4 Sources that can be used to assist community analysis

Component	Possible source
History	Local library Historical societies Local consultation (elders, etc.)
Demographics	Local government Census data Chamber of Commerce Observation
Household types and structure	Census data
Marital status	Census data
Vital statistics (births, deaths, etc.)	Government health or statistics units
Values and beliefs	Observation Community consultation

Source: Adapted from Francis et al.[36]

programme cycle, while bottom-up programmes are negotiated within and by the community, and suggest that a shift in health promotion towards empowerment requires practitioners to systematically consider community development principles within the predetermined, step-wise programme cycle.

In the PHN literature, Baillie et al.[25] argue that capacity building needs to be acknowledged as a central intervention strategy in itself, as well as a philosophical approach to PHN practice. Capacity building is a continual process that acts in parallel at each point along the public health practice cycle.

Community analysis

Understanding the attributes, nuances, cultural and historical context within the communities we work in is an important part of the intelligence required to develop PHN interventions that meet the needs of the community, and it is an important formative stage in capacity building. Community analysis also helps identify key stakeholders and target group locations and helps provide a basis for community engagement.

Table 4.4 summarises some of the data types and sources that can be used to assist community analysis.

Practice note

In many countries demographic health surveys follow a common protocol and provide data on a range of community health statistics.
  See www.measuredhs.com/aboutsurveys/dhs/start.cfm.

Key points

- Successful PHN practice involves engaging the community or population at the first stages of intervention management. Effective PHN practitioners are those that act as catalysts for community action and empower others to develop intelligent strategies to deal with identified determinants of nutrition-related health problems.
- Community development is a key strategic approach to public health capacity building and emphasises community engagement and participation, equity, empowerment and community organisation. Capacity building takes a bottom-up approach to intervention management and recognises the value of investing in social and human capital.
- Capacity building is a continual, central and interlinking strategy process that acts at each point along the public health intervention management cycle. Capacity building is a prerequisite for effective PHN intervention management such that each stage of the intervention management cycle can enhance capacity.
- 'Know thy community' is an important commandment of effective PHN intervention management. Community analysis and community engagement can provide the intelligence required and empower and motivate community members to take ownership of the issue and lead the intervention.

Useful website

www.communitybuilders.nsw.gov.au
Community building is about people from the community, government and business taking the steps to find solutions to issues within their communities. Coming up with their own solutions to problems that affect them, adapting what has worked elsewhere and enlisting support from government or other partners give people a sense of achievement and empowerment. Community building is based on collective participation of people, individually and as a community, who act together to create change.

This site is useful for community organisations, volunteers, policy-makers, academics, community leaders and all those involved in government and business. The emphasis is on how to do things, and includes checklists on what community building is; how to use and interpret statistics; group work techniques; managing conflict; how to consult young people; funding sources; sustainable urban design; and partnerships with community and business. Most of the resources are Australian, but some overseas material is also included.

Chapter 5

Step 2: Problem analysis

Objectives

By the end of this chapter you should be able to:

1. Identify sources of qualitative and quantitative PHN intelligence.
2. Describe methods of collecting and analysing qualitative and quantitative PHN intelligence.
3. Apply problem analysis techniques to identify PHN problems.
4. Understand and explain the importance of problem analysis in a PHN intervention management.

Practical Public Health Nutrition, first edition. Roger Hughes and Barrie M. Margetts. Published 2011 by Blackwell Publishing Ltd. © 2011 Roger Hughes and Barrie M. Margetts.

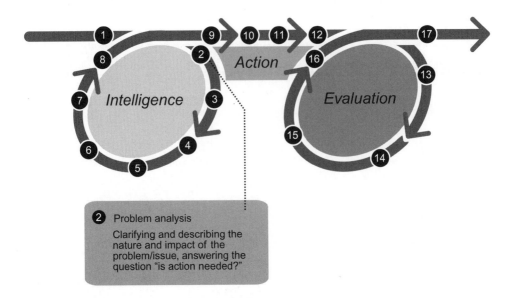

2 Problem analysis

Clarifying and describing the nature and impact of the problem/issue, answering the question "is action needed?"

Introduction

The basic premise of the problem analysis step is that you cannot efficiently solve a problem if you don't understand it. Trial-and-error strategy development (that is, practice that involves doing interventions without first understanding what needs to be done, or 'poking in the dark') may eventually hit the mark and be effective, but it is likely to be inefficient. In other words trial-and-error strategy development may improve with time because we learn from our mistakes, but takes time and wastes limited resources. Developing solutions to population-based nutrition problems (for diverse topics such as obesity or food insecurity) is that much more difficult if there is a dearth of intelligence that can be used to define specifically the problem at hand and focus attention on solutions. Problem analysis is a step in the analytical stage of the intervention bi-cycle that helps specify the nature of PHN problems.

Public health intelligence

Conducting a problem analysis involves using a variety of intelligence sources. Intelligence refers to the various types and sources of information required to accurately assess a population's need or problem and inform efficient decision-making about solutions. Intelligence is a more broad-ranging and inclusive concept than *evidence* as traditionally used in the clinical, epidemiological or research context, which usually entails evidence from randomised control trials or other reductionist or rigid research methods. Intelligence draws heavily on these sources (usually from the literature), but includes other, less normative information from sources close to the problem being addressed.

Intelligence includes information derived from consultation with:

- *the population* – those living with the problem;
- *experts* – those who have lived the research relating to the problem;
- *practitioners* – those who try to solve the problem on a daily basis.

Building on community engagement covered in the previous chapter, the term 'intelligence' recognises that there are many perspectives and contexts that need to be considered when trying to understand and effectively address a population's health problem. Such an approach to information-gathering enhances engagement and builds capacity within the community and other key stakeholders, which can further augment the successful outcomes of the intervention. It also recognises alternative sources of wisdom (such as that in the community) other than that from researchers or experts which can sometimes be biased because of a disengagement from the realities as lived by communities.

> *Public health intelligence* refers to knowledge from analysis that leads to innovative solutions and ideas generated from knowledge of the evidence base, an understanding of the problem's determinants and consultation and awareness of the contextual issues at a local population level. It may include information and data from:

- epidemiological studies;
- assessment of the various types of community needs (needs assessment);
- intervention research (what solutions have worked elsewhere);
- experiential learning (what has been learnt from the experience of doing);
- subjective or formative insights to issues and problems (from community and stakeholder consultation).

Intelligence-gathering in the PHN intervention management bi-cycle involves steps 1–8 (the intelligence stage). These steps aim to ensure that an adequate investigation of the available intelligence is conducted prior to spending time and resources on actions. Problem analysis and intelligence-gathering aids the development of successful strategies and helps to prevent inappropriate or ineffective action.

What is problem analysis?

Problem analysis involves conducting a detailed assessment of the population's needs and/or problems. Such analysis includes examination of both general population issues and the specific, nutrition-related health problem. Efforts to understand the problem help ensure that interventions are developed based on intelligence rather than assumptions, professional opinions or knowledge from limited sources. It is also important that the knowledge used to inform decision-making is specific to the problem being addressed.

Problem analysis takes place early in the PHN intervention management bi-cycle because this information is required to effectively plan, implement and evaluate population-based nutrition interventions. The process of problem analysis builds on the activities and relationships established through the community engagement and analysis step of the bi-cycle, and provide the foundation for later steps of stakeholder analysis and determinant analysis.

The term 'needs assessment' is commonly used in intervention management cyclical frameworks and is considered a vital component of effective programmes. In the PHN intervention management bi-cycle, the needs assessment is encapsulated in two stages: problem analysis (step 2) and determinant analysis (step 4). The types of intelligence that will give a good indication of the nutrition needs of a community and provide an essential foundation for intervention or service planning investigates the following questions:

- What is the nature and characteristics of communities?
- How are current services and initiatives responding to illness and promoting population health?
- Are there any gaps in services?
- What environmental changes are required for better health?[37]

These questions refer to both health and non-health services that impact on health.

The information collected from these four questions and the problem analysis should be adequate for use in:

- the allocation of resources;
- planning services and health promotion initiatives;
- setting priorities;
- reallocating funds and services.[37]

Types of need

There are two understandings of what constitutes a need:

1   A subjective concept judged by an expert or professional and influenced by whether a need can be met.
2   An objective and universal concept which is a fundamental human right.[29]

A widely used taxonomy classifies four types of need: felt, expressed, comparative and normative. Each classification provides useful information to aid priority-setting and health service planning.[38] Table 5.1 outlines the four types of social need.

Being able to describe the problem/issue you are dealing with clearly and succinctly is a prerequisite for effective intervention management because it helps focus the strategic approaches used. It is important that your team (partners, community, etc.) agree on what the problem is.

Conducting a problem analysis

The process of conducting a problem analysis can vary in terms of timing, breadth and research technique; depending on staff, financial and other resource limitations. Some general considerations for conducting a problem analysis include:

- *Participation* – involves identified participants/stakeholders (community and other key stakeholders) as much as possible. Ask about issues and assets through interviews, surveys and focus groups.
- *Time* – a problem analysis takes time to properly assess the situation from all angles. Assist the process by collecting information from readily available sources and prepare a clear agenda and supporting documents for meetings arranged to examine the data summaries.
- *Financial and other resources* – problem analysis is a discrete step that provides a clear product and useful information to many people living or working in the community. Use this opportunity to seek additional funding or sponsorship and build partnerships with those with expertise in gathering or interpreting data.
- *Data gathering* – consider and include strengths, capabilities and resources, as well as deficits and problems. Gather and analyse a variety of data by:

Table 5.1   Four types of social need

Type of need	Definition	Advantages/Disadvantages
Felt	What members of the community say they want or desire. Community consultation and development are used to assess this form of need.	Does not provide an accurate picture because: • People may limit reporting needs to what they think they can have. • People may only report needs that they think you are interested in. • Those consulted may not be representative of the community. • Interest groups can easily influence felt needs. A vital component of determining felt need is identifying the right community members to consult.
Expressed	Needs identified by demand on health services by a particular service, e.g. waiting lists for dietitian, etc.	Even more limited as an indicator of need than felt need because demand can only be expressed for available services. Can be misinterpreted, e.g. waiting lists for dental surgery may reflect a need for dental health promotion rather than more dentists.
Comparative	Arises when one community lacks services that are provided in another, similar community.	Comparative need draws on the precedent set in other regions. Problematic in that it is based on the assumption that the service provided by the area in comparison was the right response to the problem.
Normative	Refers to the needs of a community defined by experts who judge the community on the basis of their own experience.	Often carries the assumption that it is value-free and beyond reproach; expert-defined. Can be paternalistic and misleading, depending on the values of the experts. Epidemiological data are often used to define normative needs.

Source: Adapted from Bradshaw.[38]

– listing methods for collecting data and breaking the methodology down into identifiable steps;
– determining who already has useful, accessible information or data;
– seeking to continually identify and fill data gaps.

Table 5.2 summarises various methods of collecting population health intelligence and highlights the strengths, limitations and applications of each approach.

Table 5.2   Sources and methods of collecting population health intelligence

Approach	Description	Strengths	Limitations	Applications
National Statistics Age- and cause-specific mortality; life expectancy, morbidity/ hospital activity use of services	Nationally collected data	Covers whole country		Cause-specific trends over time, variation in rates by key indicators to identify at-risk groups
International and national data on food expenditure	FAO Food Balance Sheet or National Household Budget Survey data	Trends in food patterns over time	Expenditure, not actual consumption; no breakdown by age or gender	Monitoring trends over time and comparison internationally
National quality of life/ household surveys (may include regular health survey, covering diet and activity, as well as knowledge, attitudes and beliefs); National Health Survey (compilation of routine data)	Annual or less frequent surveys of a nationally representative sample	Nationally representative sample	For nutritional measures indicators limited by constraints of methodology; sample size may limit accuracy of local level estimates	Monitoring trends; comparison
National nutrition surveys	National sample, may be surveyed every ten years or more	Detailed assessment of nutrition	Expensive and not surveyed frequently so data may not reflect latest patterns; cross-check with indicator measures in national surveys	Assess proportion of population not meeting requirements; more detailed exploration of associations

Table 5.2 *Continued*

Approach	Description	Strengths	Limitations	Applications
Review of literature Published programme reports Scientific studies	Reported experience of others	Draws on proven approaches	Studied population may be different from yours	Apply scientific findings in design of programmes
Interview/ discussion (all types)	Qualitative data	Broad, rich views	Time-consuming	Expand understanding of issues and values
Key informant interviews	Structured and/ or open-ended, 20–60 minutes	In-depth understanding, build relationship	Can be biased if you include only those 'friendly' to your cause	Community values and priorities
Focus group discussion	1–2 hours, invited individuals, skilled moderator	Wide range of ideas and reactions	Time-consuming to transcribe data; responses may be influenced by other group members	Designing new or revising programmes, materials or approaches
Community leadership analysis	Interview identified 'leaders'	Learn power structure of community	Scheduling time with important people	Use when external support is important to success
Community Advisory Board	Ongoing group or purposefully selected representatives	They have understanding of programme goals and community needs	May have own agenda	Wide range of input over time
Participant observation	Observe as member of community	Reality-based	Observer must be culturally aware	Understand community practices
Inventory resources	Directory of all nutrition-related services	Recognise referral network and partners to share challenges	May not address effectiveness or appropriate access	Identify service gaps and redundancy

Different methodological approaches to gather intelligence for problem assessment

Qualitative and quantitative data sources

Two main paradigms of research analysis can be used to assist problem analysis. Qualitative and quantitative analysis. These are summarised in the box.

Qualitative research

Although qualitative research does not produce hard figures, it has a sound methodological and theoretical basis and can provide trustworthy and useful data:

- *Bottom-up research* – a tool used for seeing and understanding the world through the eyes of others.
- Need to know the community – local knowledge helps.
- Examples of qualitative techniques:
  - participant observation;
  - in-depth interviews;
  - nominal group techniques;
  - focus groups;
  - Delphi technique.

Advantages

- Can identify previously unrecognised needs.
- Incorporates a large number of approaches with potential to general a lot of information.
- Less restrictive in its investigation.
- Doing qualitative research can be an end in itself – a community learning experience.

Disadvantages

- Qualitative research should not be reported as if it were quantitative.
- Qualitative research data should be presented in a balanced manner or they can be misleading.
- Does not provide representative data.

Quantitative research

Examples include:

- Cross-sectional surveys.
- Cohort studies.
- ABS census data collections.
- Data from other organisations:
  - epidemiological;
  - hospital data, etc.

Advantages

- Can be representative of large groups and so can derive inference to whole populations.

- Can be used to dispel myths.
- Can yield statistical information from which needs can be inferred.
- Useful for testing hunches/hypotheses.
- Can assist with broad comparisons with other areas.
- Can help assess demographic change over time.
- Can be easily presented and understood
- Can be used to support arguments for new programmes.

Practice note

Brief example: Problem analysis intelligence plan
Problem and context

High consumption of unhealthy food (high fat and energy content) by employees at Springfield nuclear power plant, contributing to high obesity rates.

Proposed intelligence gathering process

In order to understand food consumption behaviour the following information collection processes are planned:

- *Literature review:* to identify data from research on consumption, determinants of workplace food consumption, intervention research concerning what has been done and what works. Establish evidence (or logic) linking workplace food consumption and health impacts.
- *Local target group consultation:* conduct face-to-face interviews with target group on leaving workplace canteen to explore motivations for takeaway food consumption and identify preferences and awareness.
- *Workplace food supply retailer group consultation:* conduct interview to identify retailer motivations, practices and beliefs re : healthy food options.
- *Mapping exercise of geographical location of food outlets in vicinity of workplace:* to identify access issues.
- *Consult community health workers and OH&S staff:* Use existing networks to explore existing services related to issue, and potential collaborators.

SWOT analysis

As a device to focus problem analysis, a SWOT analysis identifies the *strengths, weaknesses, opportunities* and *threats* of the leading organisation, community and external stakeholders and is often an effective way to identify support and potential stumbling blocks for change.[39] A SWOT analysis considers both the internal strengths and weaknesses and the external opportunities and threats. A SWOT analysis encourages a comprehensive examination of the trends and forces in the environment and consideration of their possible effects on the organisation of the programme.[40]

The *internal* SWOT analysis objectively evaluates the resources (people, facilities, etc.), competencies and culture of the organisation; the effectiveness of the current mission and strategy; and indicators of past performance. The *external* assessment includes exploration of political, economic, social, educational and technological forces and trends, along with demographic and epidemiological trends and data.

It is important to note that the SWOT analysis not only includes nutrition and health issues, but also explores unfolding political, social and technological and other forces that may influence the mission, strategy, goals and operations of the organisation and community in the future. The acquisition of additional sources of intelligence is likely to be required for a thorough SWOT analysis.

A SWOT analysis is completed in four steps:

1   *Internal analysis* – examine the capabilities and strengths of the organisation and community (management, programme delivery, financial).
2   *External analysis* – identify the main points in the environment that pose opportunities for the organisation, community and intervention, and those that pose threats or obstacles to implementing the intervention.
3   Enter the information collected in steps 1 and 2 into a grid:

	Positive	Negative
Internal assessment	*Strengths*	*Weaknesses*
External assessment	*Opportunities*	*Threats*

4   Use this information to succinctly define the problem and develop intervention strategies.[39]

Applying the intelligence and analysis results

The introduction section or rationale for an intervention plan (see the intervention template in appendix 1) is largely a description of your need, problem and determinant analysis. The problem analysis should include a process of intelligence- gathering and analysis that enables you to use this intelligence to answer the questions in Table 5.3.

Practice note

When writing submissions or plans for funding/resource allocation, it is essential to succinctly but thoroughly describe the problem your intervention plan or proposal will address. On reading your problem description, a reviewer should be very clear about the 'what?', 'who?' and 'what if?' questions relevant to the problem. They need to be convinced that it is a real problem that needs support and resources. Problem analysis should lead to a description of intelligence that makes it clear that doing nothing about the problem is unacceptable or unsustainable. If problem analysis does not lead to this sort of description, then it probably isn't a problem worth addressing (i.e. the implications of doing nothing are minimal).

Table 5.3 Questions to be answered in the problem analysis process

	Question	Example
PROBLEM DATA	What is the problem?	This should isolate the health outcome you want or need to improve or protect, e.g. *A high rate of obesity related to premature mortality and morbidity*
	Who does it affect and how many are affected?	This should focus on who is most affected by this problem and how far the problem is distributed in a population, e.g. *Obesity is most prevalent among middle-aged males with low education levels*
IMPACT	What are the attributable effects, costs, etc. of the problem (premature morbidity, burden of disease, etc.)?	This should explain the opportunity for prevention and the significant impact prevention can have, e.g. *The health and social burden of obesity is ~95% attributable to dietary and physical activity behaviours and therefore is almost entirely preventable.*
	What are the consequences of doing nothing?	This should describe an argument for action rather than maintaining the status quo. This is the 'hook' or shock statement in the introduction to an intervention management submission/plan and should clearly articulate the consequences of inaction, e.g. *A failure to implement strategies that increase physical activity and fruit and vegetable intake and reduce intake of energy-dense foods will result in an increased burden of disease, increased health care costs and reduced workforce productivity, etc.*
SUPPORT	Are the issues important to community members? Is there community support? Are resources available to support addressing the issue?	This should outline the community engagement that has occurred and the support from the community in taking action to address the problem. Any resources that have already been committed to action on this problem should also be included, e.g. *Community interviews and surveys showed that 72% of community residents were concerned about and want action to change the increasing rates of obesity, particularly among middle-aged men who are role models for their children, etc.*

Key points

- Problem analysis involves conducting a detailed assessment of the population's need or problem. A problem analysis involves using a variety of public health intelligence sources, such as information derived from consultation with the population, experts and practitioners, as well as research and epidemiological literature.
- Problem analysis occurs early in the PHN intervention management bi-cycle because this information is required to effectively plan, implement and evaluate population-based nutrition interventions.
- Undertaking a problem analysis involves gathering and analysing a range of qualitative and quantitative data to identify: (a) what the key issues are for the community or population; (b) what the impact of these issues; and (c) what level of support and resources are available to take action to address these issues.

Chapter 6

Step 3: Stakeholder analysis and engagement

Objectives

By the end of this chapter you should be able to:

1. Explain why stakeholder analysis and engagement are important in PHN intervention management.
2. Identify stakeholders relevant to PHN issues and problems.
3. Apply stakeholder analysis techniques to understand the agendas of stakeholders.
4. Demonstrate how stakeholder analysis assists with PHN problem resolution and successful intervention management

Practical Public Health Nutrition, first edition. Roger Hughes and Barrie M. Margetts. Published 2011 by Blackwell Publishing Ltd. © 2011 Roger Hughes and Barrie M. Margetts.

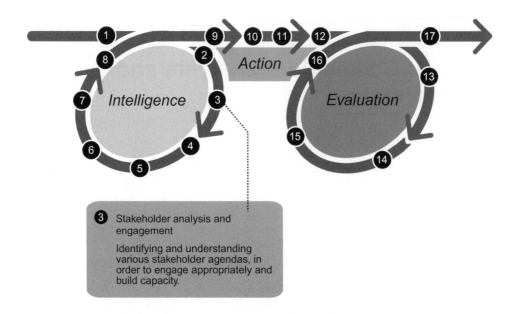

Stakeholder analysis and engagement

3 Stakeholder analysis and engagement

Identifying and understanding various stakeholder agendas, in order to engage appropriately and build capacity.

Introduction

There is increasing recognition of the central role of stakeholders – individuals, groups and organisations – who have an interest, or stake, in and the potential to influence the actions and aims of a project or policy direction.[41] By collecting and analysing data on stakeholders, an understanding of who will be affected or concerned by the identified PHN issue can be reached. It also enables an assessment of interest and influence in developing solutions and identifies stakeholder alliances or conflicts that can assist with managing stakeholder relationships throughout the intervention. Stakeholder engagement builds on the work already achieved by community engagement and uses these relationships with community stakeholders to identify other stakeholders of relevance to the identified PHN issue. *It is a critical stage in developing capacity building partnerships, which are so often important in developing effective population-based interventions.*

Stakeholder analysis is a critical formative step in intervention management because it:

- helps identify existing capacity (interest, influence, support, resources, etc.);
- identifies opposition to change (those who have a vested interest in resisting intervention strategies); and
- focuses partnership development efforts so important in building capacity to effectively deliver effective and sustainable interventions.

A failure to identify, analyse and engage stakeholders risks compromising intervention success.

A stakeholder analysis is best undertaken during the intelligence phase of intervention management as stakeholder participation throughout the process can greatly increase capacity to achieve successful and sustainable intervention outcomes. This chapter focuses on introducing the concept and process of stakeholder analysis. As the third step in PHN intervention management bi-cycle, it builds on the contextual considerations already addressed in stages 1 and 2.

Stakeholder analysis should consider the following questions:

1 Who does the problem affect most?
2 Which section of this problem-affected group is most likely to be able to change?
3 Who will be resistant to change or difficult to engage?
4 Who is in a position to help bring about change to address the problem?
5 Who has a vested interest in maintaining the status quo (i.e. no change)?
6 Who wants to see the problem addressed (what community support for change is there and who are these supporters)?
7 What government or organisational jurisdictions or responsibilities are involved or should be involved?

Why stakeholder engagement?

The purpose of stakeholder engagement is to make sure that anybody who can stop or facilitate an intervention or facilitate successful delivery should be consulted, or their views ascertained and addressed or dismissed, before the intervention begins in the planning stage. There is increasing recognition of the central role of stakeholders – individuals, groups and organisations – who have an interest, or stake, in and the potential to influence the actions and aims of a project or policy direction.[41]

By collecting and analysing data on stakeholders, an understanding of who will be affected or concerned by the identified PHN issue, as well as their level of *interest* and *influence* in developing solutions, can be gained. Stakeholder analysis and engagement builds on the work already achieved from community engagement and uses these relationships with community stakeholders to identify additional internal and external stakeholders of relevance to the identified PHN issue.

Stakeholder analysis

Stakeholder analysis is the process of identifying and generating knowledge about the key stakeholders around an intervention.[41] Understanding the behaviour, interests, interrelations and intentions can be used to assess the influence, resources and effect these stakeholders can have on the viability of the intervention. Stakeholder analysis includes both winners and losers, and those involved or excluded from the decision-making processes. It even involves identifying stakeholders who may be barriers to change, so that they can be managed or neutralised.

A stakeholder analysis can be used to inform intervention planning, implementation and evaluation. Once the key PHN issues have been identified, stakeholder analysis is used to identify who is or will be affected by these issues and their level of interest and influence. Identifying stakeholders and their interests in the issues can assist with managing current or potential conflict of interest, or assist with the development of stakeholder 'coalitions' of intervention sponsorship, ownership or cooperation. A stakeholder analysis is best undertaken during the intelligence phase of intervention management as stakeholder participation throughout the process can greatly increase the capacity to achieve intervention success. The process of stakeholder engagement and participation assists the development of a clearer understanding of the situation surrounding the PHN issue, including the political, economic, environmental and social factors. Stakeholders of relevance may come from the government sector, private sector, health-related sector, non-health services sector and of the community sector.

Considerations for stakeholder analysis

As stakeholder analysis is the third stage in the PHN intervention management bi-cycle, many of the contextual considerations for the analysis may have been addressed. However, to ensure a successful stakeholder analysis is achieved, the key preparatory considerations are outlined below:

- *Understanding the culture and context* – To interact with stakeholders and collect information successfully it is important to understand the culture and context of the various stakeholders, and how best to approach and interact with them. For example, fruit and vegetable retailers may work long hours and have very early morning starts and may not be well-educated or competently literate. Failure to explore the cultural and communication constraints can affect the success of analysis and consultation. Liaison with key informants is recommended when dealing with new stakeholders.

- *Knowing the level of analysis* – The level of analysis (local, regional, national or international) influences how data are collected and who to consider as key stakeholders. The level of analysis should be determined from the problem analysis and issue identification.
- *Being practical about the extent of analysis* – The time-line and scope of the intervention, including resource limitations, frequently determines the scope of analysis. It is important to be inclusive yet pragmatic when identifying the number of stakeholders and interests.
- *Identifying the analysis team* – Analysis can be conducted by an individual or a team. A team can provide a more objective perspective of stakeholders, while an individual can ensure a consistent, more reliable approach. Ideally, an individual should be supported by a group, who can assist by identifying unfounded assumptions. Analysers may be insiders directly involved with the project or outsiders (i.e. outside the intervention). Insiders may have vested interests or strong opinions about stakeholders which may conflict with the objective process, while familiarity with cultural modes can add strength. A mixed team of insiders and outsiders provides the most valuable analysis.[42]

Practice note

Stakeholder analysis is usually done by the intervention team behind the scenes, as it involves analysis (sizing up) of key players in order to identify partners who will act to enable intervention development and implementation or to identify opponents who will act as barriers to action and change. It is worth the effort to think clearly through this process so that you identify the right stakeholders to '*work with*' and those to '*manage out*'.

Conducting the stakeholder analysis

The process and duration of identifying and engaging stakeholders can vary according to the level and complexity of the issue.

Identification

Identification of stakeholders can involve:

1   considering different components of an intervention to identify relevant organisations and individuals;

2   a review of secondary sources of data, such as published and unpublished reports, literature, policy statements or positions on the issue, etc. (more common in national or international issues);
3   awareness of relevant stakeholders (more common in clearly defined or local issues);
4   asking key stakeholders to identify other important players ('snowballing') who have or could have considerable influence in this issue.

Engagement

The best way to approach stakeholders depends on their interest in the issue or their perception of the individual/organisation that is approaching them. Stakeholders need to be assured of the value of their participation and how it will assist their organisational or individual goals.

Engagement may involve:

1   *Direct communication* – From the intervention team.
2   *Referral from a powerful stakeholder* – An introductory letter/phone call/email from a powerful stakeholder with follow-up from the analysis team (may facilitate acceptance, but may also influence or bias responses).
3   *Third party* – An approach by an independent researcher/organisation (may be viewed as neutral, however may not be considered important enough).

Data collection

Several forms of data collection can be used in stakeholder analysis. A mix of qualitative and quantitative data collection methods is best to understand the degree of consensus on issues while allowing for additional aspects of the issue to be raised and explored.

Possible data collection methods include:

1   *Face-to-face interviews* – Checklists, semi-structured interviews and structured self-administered questionnaires can be used to collect data from individuals or organisational representatives.
2   *Focus groups, group interviews or Delphi-style consultation* – May be used to collect data from groups.
3   *Access to additional secondary sources of data* – Internal or unpublished reports or positions, for example, as a result of stakeholder consultation.
4   *Feedback summaries of discussions with stakeholders* – May build trust and correct inaccurate reporting or qualify earlier responses.[42]

Stakeholder analysis worksheet

Who does the problem affect most?	
Who will be resistant to change or difficult to engage?	
Who is in a position to help bring about change to address the problem?	
Who has a vested interest in maintaining the status quo?	
Who wants to see the problem addressed (what community support for change is there and who are these supporters)?	
Which government or organisational jurisdictions or responsibilities are involved or should be involved?	

Organising and presenting stakeholder analysis data

There are a number of methods of categorising and analysing stakeholders in a way that clearly communicates the key points in stakeholder analysis.

Stakeholders can be categorised as one of the following:

Core	Usually part of the intervention management team (i.e. intervention leads/partners)
Involved	Frequently consulted or part of the process
Supportive	Provide some form of support
Peripheral	Need to be kept informed

These categories can be plotted against the different sectors involved/relevant to the issue or problem in a stakeholder analysis wheel (Figure 6.1).

An alternative, and sometimes complementary, process involves constructing a matrix or construct map to display the findings of your stakeholder analysis. A useful tool is the *stakeholder grid* (see Figure 6.2),[43] in which stakeholders are categorised according to their interests (low vs. high) and to their power related to the issue at hand (low vs. high).

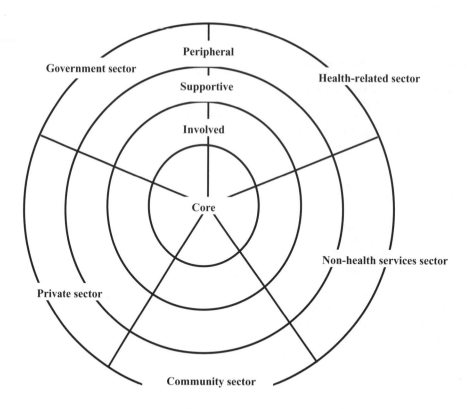

Figure 6.1   Stakeholder analysis wheel
Source: Adapted from The Health Communication Unit, *Introduction to health promotion program planning.* version 3.0, April 2001.Centre for Health Promotion, University of Toronto.

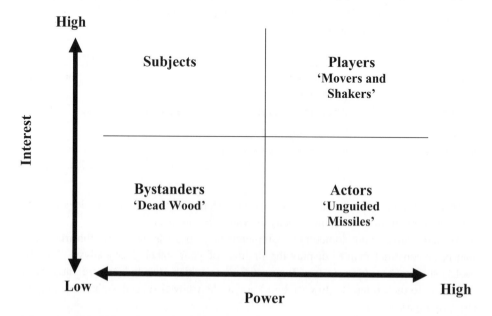

Figure 6.2   Stakeholder analysis grid
Source: Adapted from GTZ, *Capacity Building Needs Assessment (CBNA) in the Regions (version 2.0).*[43]

The matrix identifies four types of stakeholders:

1 *Actors* – Have little interest but high power; sometimes seen as 'unguided missiles' because they can unintentionally cause considerable damage.
2 *Bystanders* – Have low interest and low power; hold little influence but are not really involved.
3 *Players* – Have high interests and high power; are the 'movers and shakers' to make things happen.
4 *Subjects* – Have high interests but low power; depend on the influence and support from key players.

The use of explicit criteria for calculating scores and making assessments can reduce biases. Results from quantitative data with stakeholders (Likert scales or preferential ranking) is another way of obtaining and making stakeholder assessments.

When reviewing and applying the stakeholder findings it is useful to focus on the ultimate aim of successful implementation of the intervention and consider strategies to manage stakeholders with conflicts of interest or those with strong opposition, but high influence to the intervention. Stakeholders with substantial resources but neutral positions are important and strategies for how to mobilise those resources should be considered. Developing clear strategic alliances between stakeholders with both high interest and high influence should also be targeted.[42]

Stakeholder analysis – an example

The following extract of a stakeholder analysis exercise by Tim Lobstein in an article on childhood obesity in *SCN News* provides an example of how a stakeholder analysis grid can be used. Figure 6.3 illustrates the various stakeholders in the context of obesity, using a stakeholder analysis grid.

Stakeholder involvement – key points relating to childhood obesity

- The commercial sector has a major role and stake in the production of the obesogenic environment.
- The various views of different stakeholders may lead to challenges to the scientific basis and strength of evidence underlying any suggested policy proposals.
- Policy-makers may find it hard to support policies which limit, for example, commercial freedom or personal choice without compelling evidence of their benefit.
- Until such evidence becomes available, precautionary activities need to be undertaken based on the best available evidence supported by a consensus of scientific opinion. In this respect, professional practitioners with expertise in child obesity and related health problems play a significant role.
- It is valuable to look at the role of the stakeholders in the policy arena relevant to over-weight and obesity and to identify their characteristics. It is, for example, possible to list several of the interested parties (e.g. parents, school staff, environmental planners, food companies, advertising agencies, government ministries) and to place them on a multidimensional map which helps identify their relative position and the scope for change.

- When such a mapping exercise is undertaken it can reveal useful information for those trying to influence policy. For example, in Figure 6.3 the general trend of the scatter of data points is from top left to bottom right, i.e. the data indicate that those with the greatest influence are either neutral with regard to diet or interested in making it unhealthy. Conversely, those with the greatest interest in improving children's diets appear to have the least influence on policy.
- In order to influence policy and to restructure the graph in favour of healthier children:
    - we need to strengthen the influence of those who are currently in the top left corner of the graph;
    - we need to reduce the influence or alter the relatively negative influence of those who are currently in the lower right hand part of the graph, by finding incentives for them to change their interests so that they support healthier diets;
    - we need to make those with the most influence on policy (suggested in this graph as being national presidents, treasury secretaries) to become more interested in the promotion of healthier diets by showing the economic damage that obesity may cause and by increasing the political pressure for action.

Source: Adapted from Lobstein.[44]

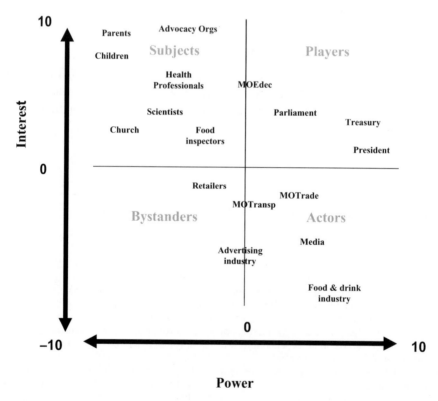

Figure 6.3   Stakeholder analysis – obesity
Source: Adapted from Lobstein.[44]

Stakeholder engagement

Once stakeholders have been identified, categorised and described, the next step is to consider strategies for engaging with those stakeholders your analysis has identified as being most useful and relevant to your intervention. Usually the most effective and practical approach is to contact stakeholders directly and invite them to partner in managing the intervention as a *core, involved, supportive or peripheral* stakeholder, depending on how involved you want them to be or how involved they want to be.

Engaging stakeholders in decision-making

If we are serious about engaging stakeholders and building capacity for effective PHN action, it is vital that the management or governance structure of the intervention is identified and agreed. The objective of intervention governance is essentially about shared decision-making to manage the project throughout its life, including the realisation of intervention deliverables, high productivity and quality output and appropriate risk management.[43]

Intervention management structures can sometimes give rise to conflict with regard to accountability and reporting, particularly when the governance structure does not reflect operational line management structures. It is therefore very important that all players know and agree with how the intervention governance structure will operate. Intervention activities should be managed through the intervention management structure, while operational activities should be managed through existing line management structures. The distinction between these two types of activities, intervention and normal business should be clearly conveyed to assist with defining accountability and reporting arrangements.[43]

Including key stakeholders on decision-making committees

An intervention management committee or steering committee is often crucial for intervention success, particularly for larger interventions. Steering committee members play an important role in the intervention, both individually and collectively. The primary function of a steering committee is to take responsibility for the business associated with an intervention, ultimately ensuring delivery of intervention activities and appropriate risk management (ensuring issues are adequately addressed and kept under control).

If management committees are to work effectively, the right people must be involved. Management committee appointment should be based on an assessment of individual skills and attributes rather than on formal roles, and members should maintain membership even if their role within an organisation changes.

A key factor in selecting individuals for decision-making committees is to be sure that their interests are vested in the success of the intervention. This insight depends on thorough stakeholder analysis.

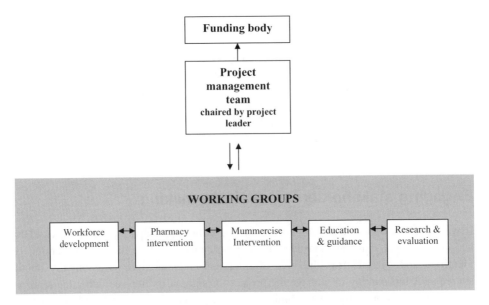

Figure 6.4   Intervention governance model for a medium-sized multi-strategy project

It may be necessary to develop Terms of Reference to which the steering committee sign off to ensure all members are aware of their roles and responsibilities of being part of the steering committee for the intervention.

In practice the intervention management committee responsibilities involve five main functions:

1 *Approval of changes to the intervention and its supporting documentation* – Including intervention priorities and objectives, budget, deliverables, schedule amendments and risk management strategies.

2 *Monitoring and review of the intervention* – Including reviewing the status of the intervention at the end of each phase to determine whether the team should progress.

3 *Providing assistance to the intervention when required* – Including being active advocates of the intervention and helping facilitate broad support for it, facilitating communication with stakeholder groups, illustrating intervention benefits and contributing individual knowledge or experience.

4 *Resolving intervention conflicts in resource allocation, output quality or level of stakeholder commitment* – While the project manager should be able to deal with most conflicts, there may be occasions when the management committee are required to help resolve disputes.

5 *Formal acceptance of intervention deliverables* – The management committee should formally review and accept project outputs and are therefore required to have a broad understanding of the intervention and approach employed by the intervention team.[43]

A steering/management committee should meet regularly throughout the course of the intervention to keep track of the progress of the intervention and address any issues that may arise. The project manager should attend these meetings to be a source of information for the committee and to be informed about the committee decisions.

The management committee has responsibility for the intervention until the deliverables and outcomes have been achieved, which may not occur until after the project team have completed their involvement.

Figure 6.4 is an example of an intervention governance model for a medium-scale intervention which may be useful to include in the intervention management committee terms of reference and implementation plan.

In this multi-partner, multi-strategy community intervention, a project management team (PMT) composed of core stakeholders (~10 individuals representing key partner organisations/jurisdictions) met fortnightly to monitor project implementation and share decision-making and information. Day-to-day implementation responsibility and decision-making have been delegated to working groups, each with separate, defined implementation budgets and plans, in regular communication with the project leader and other members via regular PMT meetings.

Key points

- Stakeholders are individuals, groups and organisations who have an interest in the issue under consideration, are affected by the issue or have an influence on intervention implementation.
- Stakeholder analysis is the process of identifying and generating knowledge about the key stakeholders of an intervention. Collecting and analysing data on stakeholders can create an understanding of who will be affected or concerned by the identified PHN issue, who is interested and will influence the development of solutions to the issue.
- A stakeholder analysis can be used to inform intervention planning, implementation and evaluation. Once the key PHN issues have been identified, stakeholder analysis is used to recognise who is or will be affected by these issues, as well as their level of interest and influence.
- Once identified, categorised and described, stakeholders need to be strategically engaged in the intervention management process.

Chapter 7

Step 4: Determinant analysis

Objectives

On completion of chapter you should be able to:

1. Identify proximal and contributory determinants of PHN problems.
2. Describe causal and associative relationships between determinants of PHN problems.
3. Ascertain intervention points based on an analysis of determinant sequencing and causal flows.

Practical Public Health Nutrition, first edition. Roger Hughes and Barrie M. Margetts. Published 2011 by Blackwell Publishing Ltd. © 2011 Roger Hughes and Barrie M. Margetts.

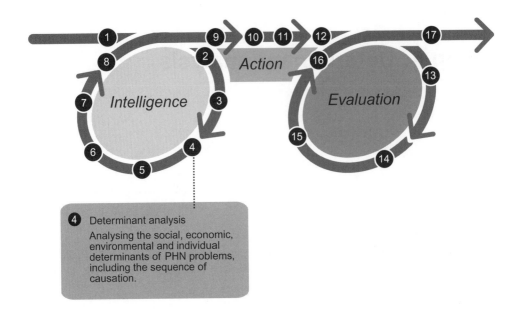

4 Determinant analysis

Analysing the social, economic, environmental and individual determinants of PHN problems, including the sequence of causation.

Introduction

The basic assumption that underpins determinant analysis as a stage in the analysis phase of the intervention bi-cycle is that problems cannot efficiently be addressed without understanding their causes. Most problems or issues we have to deal with in PHN practice are not random events but have multiple causes or determinants. Determinant analysis is consistent with the *upstream* strategy focus explicit in preventative approaches to health. Identifying determinants helps to focus strategies so that they change *upstream* the factors that lead to *downstream* outcomes (see the river of prevention analogy in Chapter 3).

Analysing determinants

Public health practice is concerned with identifying, modifying and evaluating change in the determinants (causes) of health and health problems. Determinant analysis involves identifying the factors affecting health (or a related problem) and reviewing the linkages or relationships among these factors. Determinant analysis recognises that problems have multiple causes and that identification of causal relationships is important for strategy section and prioritisation. A detailed understanding through rigorous and inclusive analysis of the determinants of a health problem is essential for effective action at a community or population level. Determinant analysis is an extension of problem analysis, community and stakeholder engagement. It applies the intelligence collected about the problem to identify and analyse the causes of the specific population nutrition problem.

Considering the socio-ecological determinants of the identified population nutrition problem is a critical analytical and conceptual exercise in the formative stages of designing preventative interventions. Various models, based on the socio-ecological approach to health, exist to assist with determinant identification and classification (such as the *precede–proceed* model). The use of classification models that characterise determinants by their effect, level and causal link is another logical approach which enables intervention points to be selected based on an analysis of determinant sequencing and causal flows.[45]

Practice note

It may well be that the causal pathway identified in determinant analysis is not linear. The logic, however, is that there is likely to be a long sequence of events leading to the current situation. If we are to address a problem now and prevent it in the future, we need to be able to trace this pathway and identify the key factors that are amenable to change and then change them.

One of the useful models for systematically exploring and understanding the determinants of a problem is the *precede–proceed model*.[46] The model focuses on identifying the subset of factors that need to be addressed by the intervention, premised on the

Table 7.1 Precede–proceed model – determinants of physical activity

Determinant category	Determinant description
Predisposing factors	Attitudes Expected health and other benefits Intention to exercise Self-motivation Past participation High risk of heart disease Perceived effort
Enabling/disabling factors	Income/socio-economic status Opportunities to exercise Time Mood disturbance Perceived level of health or fitness Self-efficacy for exercise Perceived access to facilities
Reinforcing factors	Social isolation Group cohesion Social support (staff/instructor) Social support (spouse/family)

Source: Adapted from Miilunpalo.[47]

socio-ecological view of health and the need for multidimensional, multi-sectoral efforts to address health problems.[47] The precede–proceed model suggests determinants that influence health behaviour can be classified as:

- *Predisposing factors* – Personal factors that influence personal motivation to change, including attitudes, values, beliefs, knowledge.
- *Enabling factors* – Facilitators or inhibitors that support or hinder change in behaviour or the environment, including societal forces or systems, resources or skills.
- *Reinforcing factors* – Factors that provide feedback and further assist, hinder or prohibit a behavioural or environmental change.

To illustrate: the precede–proceed model has been used to categorise the determinants of physical activity from 33 studies.[47] The results are shown in Table 7.1.

Characterising determinants by their effect

Not all determinants have negative effects on health outcomes. Another method for characterising determinants is to distinguish whether they have a positive or negative effect on the problem/issue under review.

- *Hazards* – Social, biomedical or behavioural determinants which pose a threat to health.

Table 7.2 Determinants by effect – fruit and vegetable intake

Determinant type	Definition	Example
Hazards and risk factors	Pose a threat to health	Hazards can be from the physical environment or social/behavioural/ biomedical: • poor availability; • poor quality; • high cost; • access and isolation.
Protective/ promoting	Provide a defence against adverse health events or are desirable and beneficial to health	Protective or promoting determinants for fruit and vegetable intake include: • high availability – schools, workplaces, corner stores; • healthy eating policy in schools/ workplaces; • high cultural value in fruit and vegetables.

Source: Adapted from NPHP.[45]

- *Protective factors* – Provide a defence against adverse health events or states, or enhance well-being.
- *Promoting factors* – Desirable and beneficial; they also play a protective role.

Occasionally, protective/promoting factors are the inverse of a hazard. For example, a poor diet and physical inactivity are hazardous; however, a healthy diet and regular physical activity can be protective and promote quality of life.[45] Table 7.2 provides an example of hazardous and protective/promoting determinants.

Characterising determinants by the type of causal link

Analysis of determinants needs to consider both proximate and contributory or distal effects. Health problems such as obesity are caused by factors that can be classified as immediate or proximate. These determinants directly impact on the problem (e.g. a sedentary lifestyles and energy-dense diet impact directly on obesity). At the same time, there may be several more distal determinants which create conditions for or increase the effect of the proximate determinant. Often it is only possible (and desirable) to act on the contributory determinants rather than the proximate cause (i.e. going upstream). Table 7.3 provides an example of proximate and contributory determinants.

Table 7.3   Determinants by causal link – fruit and vegetable intake

Determinant type	Definition	Example
Proximate DIRECT	Directly impacts on the problem	Adequate intake of fruit and vegetables is recognised as a proximate determinant for several diseases including obesity, type 2 diabetes, cancer and heart disease.
Distal/Contributory INDIRECT	Increase the effect of the proximate determinant	The tendency of an individual to consume adequate fruit and vegetables and the rate of adequate fruit and vegetable intake in the community are caused by a range of contributory determinants including: • age; • habit; • knowledge and skills; • perceptions of cost and safety.

Source: Adapted from NPHP[45] and Miller and Stafford.[48]

Characterising determinants by level

Determinants of health occur at two levels: the *specific* and the *social and environmental*. Specific determinants relate to downstream health events more closely related to individual causes of ill health and encompass both behavioural and biomedical factors. Social and environmental determinants are broader, upstream factors external to the individual. Social and environmental determinants can have either a hazardous or protective effect on health.[45] Strong networks of support, for example, may act as a buffer against the stresses caused by job loss. Both social/environmental and specific determinants can have a proximate or contributory effect. For example, an economic recession may lead to an individual losing her job. The *proximate* effect may be anxiety and an adverse physiological response to the stress, whereas the *contributory* effect may be less money to buy adequate fruit and vegetables which, over time, will have physiological consequences. Table 7.4 provides an example of specific and social and environmental determinants.

Figure 7.1, a hypothetical and largely incomplete determinant analysis diagram, illustrates the relationship between distal and proximal determinants, and the implicit causal logic.

The example of obesity illustrates some simple analytical distinctions which could be made to arrive at a comprehensive understanding of the nutrition-related determinants of this health problem. In this case the *proximate* determinants comprise the coincidence of two *hazards*: poor or inadequate intake of fruit and vegetables, and excessive intake of energy-dense (high sugar/fat), salty foods. These hazards may in turn depend on other *contributory* determinants, such as vast promotion of energy-dense foods (*social and*

Table 7.4 Determinants by level – fruit and vegetable intake

Determinant	Definition	Example
Specific	Health events more closely associated with individual causes of ill health.	Specific determinants can be both behavioural and biomedical: • behaviour: inadequate intake of fruit and vegetables, high intake of energy-dense food; • biomedical: obesity, spina bifida (inadequate folate), recurrent infections.
Social and environmental	Broader, upstream factors external to the individual.	Broader external factors impacting on inadequate fruit and vegetable intake: • availability; • quality and price; • promotion.

Both specific and social and environmental determinant can have a proximate or contributory effect.

Source: Adapted from NPHP[45] and Miller and Stafford.[48]

environmental) and perceptions of the cost of fruit and vegetables (*social and environmental*).

Acting on the contributory determinants may be the best point for intervention and involve strengthening *protective* and *promotive* factors, such as reducing promotion of energy-dense foods, displaying per kilogram pricing for all foods to enable comparison between fruit and vegetables and energy-dense foods, and improving knowledge about the harmful effects of energy-dense foods and the benefits of eating more fruit and vegetables.

Practice note

When analysing determinants of a population nutrition problem, use the intelligence sources gathered during the earlier steps of community engagement, problem analysis and stakeholder engagement to inform the analysis. Include these sources in your descriptions and diagrams to inform the reader. Once the determinants have been identified and the determinant sequencing and interaction illustrated in a diagram by the project team, it is important to undertake further consultation with the community and key stakeholders. Ongoing consultation and participation ensure the intervention points most likely to be successful are selected by those affected by and capable of addressing the problem – a key capacity building strategy.

Determinant interaction and causal pathways

Isolating individual determinants and understanding how they cause a problem are useful but are not the only levels of analysis required. The interaction between determinants

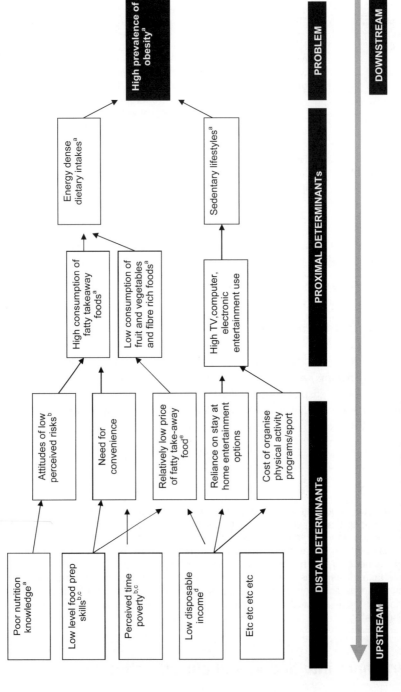

Figure 7.1 Determinants of obesity: simplified example

and how they operate in context are equally important in defining and addressing a problem. Examination of determinant sequencing and interaction avoids simplistic models of causation which can lead to simplistic and ineffective solution generation.

Remaining with adequate fruit and vegetable intake as an example, research examined some of the determinants fruit and vegetable intake in African-American women in the community of eastside Detroit.[49] The study examined two determinants – retail food store characteristics and household income – based on a variety of intelligence sources. Intelligence indicates that larger supermarket food store have better availability, superior quality and lower prices compared to smaller food stores, and that people with higher incomes tend to consume more fruit and vegetables. Store characteristics, including type and location, are considered contributory determinants which affect the proximate determinants of availability, quality and price of fruit and vegetables. While household income directly impacts on fruit and vegetable intake it can also contribute to store characteristics and location by the average level of wealth of the area. The researchers also acknowledge the impact of other contributory determinants, including age and education level, which affect several determinants and each other. This example provides an illustration of the complexity involved in understanding determinant sequencing and interaction.

Diagrammatic illustration of determinant analysis

Determinant analysis is often best presented as a diagram. A diagrammatic illustration of the food store characteristics and income as determinants of fruit and vegetable intake is present in Figure 7.2.

A diagrammatic illustration of the determinant analysis in intervention management should isolate the focus of intervention strategies. Considering Figure 7.2 and the impact store type and location have on availability, quality and cost of food a possible interven-

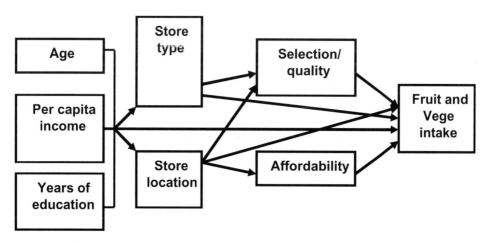

Figure 7.2   Determinant analysis diagrammatic example-fruit and vegetable intake
Source: Adapted from Zenk et al.[49]

tion point is to increase the number of or access to supermarkets in areas where there are few. Further consultation with the community and key stakeholders and progressing through the remaining steps in the intelligence section of the bi-cycle will highlight whether this intervention is achievable and will be effective.

Practice note

'A picture paints a thousand words'
Determinant analysis is often best presented as a diagram. Determinant analysis should isolate determinants that will become the focus of intervention strategies. Include a determinant analysis diagram that demonstrates the causative relationship between determinants and the problem in your project introduction/rationale section of your final submission. Include the data sources you have used to construct your determinant analysis model.

Key points

- Determinant analysis involves identifying the factors affecting health or causing a problem and reviewing the linkages or relationships among these factors. Determinant analysis recognises that problems have causes and that identification of causal relationships is an important strategy and prioritisation in PHN intervention management.
- Various models, based on the socio-ecological approach to health, are available to assist with determinant identification and classification, such as the precede–proceed model. The use of classification models that characterise determinants by their effect, level and causal link is another approach that enables intervention points to be selected, based on analysis of determinant sequencing and causal flows.
- The interaction between determinants and how they operate in the context of the setting where the nutrition-related health problem occurs is another important component of determinant analysis. Identification of determinant sequencing and interaction, and a diagrammatic illustration of the determinant analysis, are important to focus intervention points and strategies.

Chapter 8

Step 5: Capacity analysis

Objectives

On completion of chapter you should be able to:

1. Describe the role and importance of capacity building needs analysis in the PHN intervention management process.
2. Discuss the measurement issues and challenges associated with capacity building needs analysis.
3. Describe and apply the various capacity building needs analysis methods and tools to assess organisational capacity needs, training needs and capacity gaps.
4. Describe how capacity building strategies can be integrated with the PHN intervention management cycle.

Practical Public Health Nutrition, first edition. Roger Hughes and Barrie M. Margetts. Published 2011 by Blackwell Publishing Ltd. © 2011 Roger Hughes and Barrie M. Margetts.

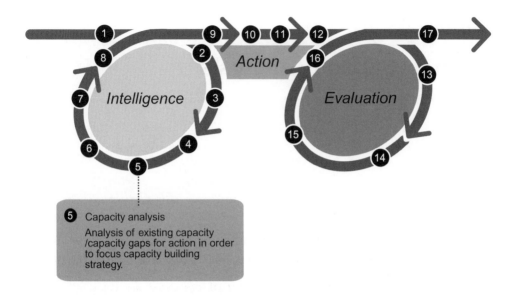

5 Capacity analysis

Analysis of existing capacity
/capacity gaps for action in order
to focus capacity building
strategy.

Introduction

A community's ability to address public health nutrition challenges (or *capacity*) is effectively determined by many factors and varies among communities and contexts. Capacity is therefore clearly of relevance to PHN practice, and intervention management in particular. Without capacity, the most innovative and brilliant ideas for interventions will not be adequately implemented or effective and will therefore fail to achieve their objectives. A failure to assess capacity and its determinants adequately in the intelligence stage of the intervention bi-cycle will increase the likelihood that existing resources (ideas, skills, commitment, political support, etc.) will not be identified and utilised, compromising intervention effectiveness and the quality of PHN practice. Analysis of capacity in the context of intervention planning is therefore critical.

What is capacity?

Capacity is a nebulous term which, simply defined, is the ability to carry out stated objectives.[50] In the context of PHN practice, capacity relates to the ability of individuals, groups, organisations, communities, the workforce and systems to perform effective, efficient and sustainable action that achieves PHN objectives.

A school community decides that overweight and obesity are problems among school children which not only affect health, but also educational and social outcomes. They decide to develop a project with broad objectives to improve the dietary and physical activity behaviours of school children. The community's capacity to deliver these objectives will depend on a number of factors (capacity determinants), including the support and leadership of the school principal and teachers, the attitudes, knowledge and skill of the teachers, funding in the school budget to support change and the facilities in the school to sell or provide healthy food choices (to name a few).

Capacity building refers to the *process* by which individuals, groups, organisations and societies increase their ability to solve problems, define objectives and understand and deal with development needs to achieve objectives in a sustainable manner.[51] As noted in Chapter 2, capacity building is an essential and central component of PHN practice. Capacity building is of relevance to many of the core functions of public health practice, including workforce development, intervention management, partnership and community development. There are several key attributes of capacity building in practice, and include the following:

- Capacity building is a continuous process.
- Capacity building contributes to better performance and is linked with the achievement of objectives.

- Capacity building works towards the establishment of a sustainable local health system where the community has the competence to address the current health problem and tackle other health issues.
- Capacity building operates at numerous levels (individual, organisational and systematic level).[52]

The capacity building literature outside public health suggests that capacity building should be an interlinked, continual process consisting of several components:

- assessment of capacity needs;
- planning of a capacity building programme;
- implementation of the capacity building activities;
- evaluation impacts of capacity building activities to restart the capacity building process.[43]

Note that in the bi-cyclic framework for intervention management described in Chapter 3, these four stages are integrated with the development and delivery of PHN interventions.

A framework for capacity building practice

Building on the work of scholars in the health promotion arena, Baillie et al.[52] have identified the domains of capacity building in PHN practice to provide a focus for assessing, planning, implementing and evaluating capacity building strategies in practice. A conceptual framework (Figure 8.1) presents these domains, showing key foundations for capacity building in PHN practice as leadership, resourcing and intelligence. Building on these layers are five strategic domains, including partnerships, organisational development, project management quality, workforce development and community development. These capacity domains are core components of the PHN competency framework, illustrating that capacity building practice is a key element of quality PHN practice and performance.

Capacity assessment for capacity building

The main use of this framework is to isolate the components of a community's capacity so that gaps can be identified, strategies focused and changes in capacity monitored and evaluated. Conducting a capacity analysis should be a fundamental element of capacity building in practice. Before beginning to build capacity within and around public health interventions, practitioners need to identify and respect the existing skills, structures, partnerships and resources, to be able to work with this capacity.[53] Capacity assessment also involves identifying and building on existing capacities at each of the various levels (individual, managerial, organisational and systematic), to enable strategy development and to establish baseline measures for capacity building evaluation.

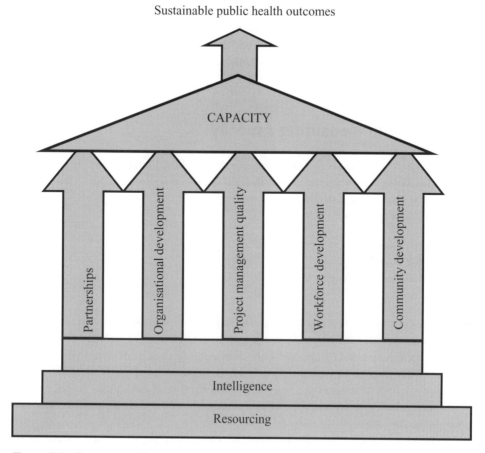

Figure 8.1   Capacity building conceptual framework

Experience elsewhere has shown that the process of assessing or measuring capacity is as important as the implementation of targeted capacity building initiatives, especially if the assessment process involves participatory group discussions, workshops and joint assessment exercises. The selection of tools and instruments must therefore be geared towards creating such discussion and learning opportunities for the members of an project team, organisation or community.[43]

Effective capacity building practice links local people with community expertise together with practitioners with technical and capacity building expertise. Such links allow for an exchange of identified and valued knowledge between groups which aids the development of trust and enhanced community engagement. Capacity analysis in itself can often lead to capacity building because it engages and empowers community stakeholders.

Interventions that are integrated into existing structures and linked to existing positions and accountability processes are more likely to be sustained. Capacity analysis ensures capacity building strategies are contextually appropriate and tailored to the specific conditions of the community/population or organisation. For successful capacity building interventions, practitioners need the ability to observe accurately, to interpret observations intelligently and impersonally, and then deliver the appropriate intervention at the appropriate time.

Challenges in measuring capacity

Building capacity to effectively implement community-based interventions is an integral part of the 'doing' of public health nutrition. The 'doing' focus on capacity building is integrally linked to and dependent on measuring capacity.

Capacity assessment serves to:

• identify a communities readiness for action;
• engage the community;
• focus strategies for capacity building;
• provide baseline data for capacity building strategy evaluation.

Assessment of capacity is required at various stages of capacity development and different measures may be necessary at each stage. Initial assessment of capacity provides the context for capacity building and identifies its possibilities and gaps. Progressive assessments monitor change in capacity at individual, organisational and systematic levels. Impact measurement assesses the amount of capacity gain at the various levels, as well as the successful elements of the capacity building strategy and their contribution to the intervention outcomes.

The method of measuring baseline capacity, changes in capacity and the benefits of capacity building on health can be challenging. A number of issues influencing measurement of capacity have been identified from Canadian health promotion capacity building experience.[54] These issues are not mutually exclusive, with many of them interacting with each other. These are not that different from measurement issues in other areas of research and evaluation. The key issues and challenges in measuring capacity are our outlined in Table 8.1.

A number of strategies to address the identified issues in measuring capacity have been suggested and outlined in Table 8.2.

Selecting tools for capacity analysis

Capacity building is contextual and bound to the specific conditions of each community, so the approach for conducting a systematic capacity analysis should take these specific conditions into account and select tools and instruments for the analysis process, which can then be adjusted to the existing conditions. Each analysis will be different and use a different mixture of diagnostic tools.[43]

Table 8.1 Issues in measuring capacity

Issues	Description
Multiple understandings of terms	Lack of consistent understanding of health promotion terminology across settings, organisations and individuals present a measurement challenge as a shared terminology cannot be assumed when exploring health promotion capacity with key informants at multiple levels of an organisation or across sectors. This issue has implications in the design and format of measurement tools, and for data analysis.
Evolving understanding of capacity	The definition and nature of capacity are evolving, thus measurement tools, particularly quantitative tools, can be lengthy and complex in order to tap into actual or potential dimensions. Respondent burden becomes an issue.
Invisibility of capacity building	Community empowerment is explicit in health promotion, which often creates a culture of invisibility around capacity building (because capacity building practitioners want the community to take ownership and credit for capacity gains and the associated outcomes, they may not communicate or promote capacity building strategies overtly). Invisibility causes difficulty in recognising, describing and measuring capacity building.
Dynamic contexts	The health system is dynamic and always seems to be threatening dramatic restructuring. Prominent contextual aspects that have influenced the measurement of capacity include: staff turnover, health system renewal, conflicting perspectives across informants within organisations, conflicting personalities within organisations and between informants and practitioners, 'turf' protection' by health workers in different departments, and organisational staff understanding and valuing the capacity building process.
Time course for change	The long-term outcome is that enhanced capacity will ultimately contribute to improved health in the population. Organisational and/or individual capacity serves as an intermediate outcome, as do enhanced health promotion and prevention skills, services and programmes. The time course for such individual or system changes is a challenge for projects with set timeframes.
Building trust and dealing with sensitive issues	It is important to develop a trusting relationship among practitioners and organisational or community representatives to ensure high quality data collection. Equally important is the longitudinal nature of the research which requires multiple connections over time. The relationships underlying these multiple connections depend on trust and are a mediating factor that should not be underestimated. The development of appropriate questions and the documenting and sharing such sensitive information without breaching confidentiality or trust pose a measurement challenge.
'Snapshot' measurements	Quantitative instruments provide a 'snapshot' in time. Qualitative interviews allow the exploration of critical events, milestones or snapshots; however, they rely on accurate and comprehensive recall, sometimes months after a particular occurrence. This can be a limitation because of recall bias.

Table 8.1   *Continued*

Issues	Description
Validity and reliability of quantitative measures	There is no gold standard against which to measure health promotion capacity. Establishing criterion validity is therefore compromised. External validity, the generalisability of findings to and across populations of subjects and settings, is difficult to attain because each project is context-specific.
Attribution for change in capacity	The process for building health promotion capacity is participatory, in that organisations and individuals who are the 'recipients' of the capacity-building interventions are integrally involved in developing, planning and evaluating the process. If the principles of participatory action and health promotion are adhered to, then 'others' take ownership and embrace the work as their own. This ownership is both a positive aspect of the process and an outcome. However, identifying both the successful elements of the capacity-building strategy and the independent contributions of the intervention becomes complex.

Source: Adapted from Ebbesen et al.[54]

Table 8.2   Strategies to address key capacity measurement issues

Strategy	Measurement issue addressed
Utilise participatory processes as intervention	Multiple understandings of terms. Evolving understanding of capacity. Building trust and dealing with sensitive issues.
Acknowledge the context	Invisibility of capacity building. Dynamic context.
Incorporate mixed methods (qualitative and quantitative)	Invisibility of capacity building. Dynamic contexts. Time course for change. Building trust and dealing with sensitive issues Snapshot measures. Validity and reliability of quantitative methods. Attribution for change in capacity
Build on previous phases of community and stakeholder engagement	Multiple understandings of terms. Building trust and dealing with sensitive issues.
Establish validity of quantitative measures	Validity and reliability of quantitative methods.
Establish trustworthiness of qualitative intelligence	Multiple understanding of terms. Evolving understanding of capacity. Time course for change. Building trust and dealing with sensitive issues. Snapshot measures

Table 8.2 *Continued*

Strategy	Measurement issue addressed
Be flexible and adaptable	Dynamic contexts. Multiple understanding of terms. Building trust and dealing with sensitive issues.
Identify intervention contributions (i.e. intervention-specific evaluations)	Attribution for change in capacity.

Source: Adapted from Ebbesen et al.[54]

Deciding on the assessment approach and the tools to be applied requires an initial examination of the contextual factors that impact on tool selection. Some of the key factors to be considered are outlined in Table 8.3.

Tools and strategies for analysing capacity

Many of the tools used in capacity analysis can draw on intelligence collected from the previous steps in the intelligence stage of the PHN intervention management bi-cycle. Capacity analysis involves building on the information collected in the community engagement and stakeholder analysis steps, and the subsequent identification and formation of the project management committee (see capacity building strategies later in this chapter).

Practice note

One of the most useful and important capacity building strategies in most PHN management situations is the development of a *project management committee*. This committee serves as a partnership or coalition of key stakeholders – usually those that you have previously engaged with and assessed as being interested and who have influence in the community. This committee becomes a system for intervention governance (decision-making, accountability, etc.), which is important for ethical and effective PHN practice.

It is important and advantageous to involve the project management committee in capacity analysis. As this group typically includes representatives from the community, key stakeholder groups and management they have an essential role in identifying capacity potential and gaps and resources to support capacity building. Working with the identified project management group members to determine the scope, responsibilities and tasks, and methodology and tools for the capacity analysis helps to enhance stakeholder commitment to and involvement in the capacity building process.

Table 8.4 lists a range of tools that have been developed to assist capacity assessment and analysis.

Table 8.3 Factors influencing the selection of capacity analysis tools

Factor	Description
Internal (self-) assessment vs. external assessment	Some of the tools and instruments can by applied by the organisation itself. Others require the use of external consultants, moderators and/or facilitators. Both approaches have their strengths and weaknesses: *Internal assessment* can be biased and subjective; however, it has a better understanding and knowledge of the organisation's culture and members. *External assessment* has less bias; however, it can miss some important aspects of an organisation if the external assessor is not given the inside information needed. Cost is another factor since external consultants or moderators are (normally) paid.
Level of assessment	The mix of instruments used for the assessment of capacity needs to capture capacity building information for all three levels of capacity (systems level, organisational level, individual level). *Not all instruments will be useful and feasible for all levels of the analysis.* (See Table 8.4. for recommended analysis tools for each level of capacity.)
Type of organisation(s)	Is the organisation public, private, for-profit or not-for-profit? Many tools and instruments for capacity assessment have been developed for a specific type of organisation. However, they can usually be adjusted to capture the characteristics and conditions of other organisations.
Comparability across organisations	Whether one wants to compare capacities across organisations or limit the capacity assessment to a single organisation can have a bearing on the selection of tools. Comparison requires the tool to measure the same capacity areas for all organisations, use the same scoring criteria and the same measurement process. Such a standardised tool might therefore be less capable of capturing the specific situation of an individual organisation.
Comparability over time	Do you intend to assess capacity over time (i.e. repeatedly) in order to observe and document the capacity changes, or is the capacity analysis a one-off exercise? Comparability over time requires consistency in method and approach, and the measurement instrument needs to be applied in the same way each time it is used. A baseline would also need to be established.
Data collection methods	Some methods are more participatory than others, some are simple, and others need specialist expertise. Data collection methods include: open, structured or semi-structured interviews with individuals, document analysis, observation, field visits and focus groups. *In most cases, a mix of several data collection methods will produce better results than the use of just one method.*
Objectivity	Measures of institutional capacity are usually subjective in relying on individual perception, analysis and judgement. They provide qualitative information, rather than quantitative data. Subjective perception of capacity can, to a certain extent, be balanced by other more empirical tools.

Table 8.3 *Continued*

Factor	Description
Quantification	Depending on the measurement tools, organisational capacity can be expressed in numbers, using ordinal scales. Note that these numbers are not absolute but relative. Combining quantitative data with qualitative descriptions can provide a better, more accurate picture of an organisation's capacity.
Practicality and efficiency	Diagnostic tools should provide useful information and not be too complicated, time-consuming or costly. In selecting tools, consider the level of effort (burden) and resources required to develop the instrument, and collect and analyse the data. Selecting only one tool can be tempting because it will be easier to use and faster (and perhaps cheaper). However, using several tools can provide richer and more comprehensive information. Using multiple tools can also help to balance their respective weaknesses.

Source: Adapted from GTZ, *Capacity Building Needs Assessment (CBNA) in the Regions (version 2.0).*[43]

Table 8.4 Level of capacity and suggested analysis tool

Level of assessment	Suggested tool
System/institutional level	Document analysis Force field analysis Focus group analysis Stakeholder analysis
Organisational level	Document analysis Organisational capacity assessment SWOT analysis Focus group discussion Stakeholder analysis
Individual level	Document analysis Focus group discussion Task and job analysis Training needs assessment

Source: Adapted from GTZ, *Capacity Building Needs Assessment (CBNA) in the Regions (version 2.0).*[43]

Document analysis

Document analysis is the systematic examination of documents to identify organisational objectives, policy mandates, resources and associated needs, potential and challenges. The analysis should be a critical examination rather than a simple description of the documents. Document analysis can provide insight into systematic, organisational or individual positions on an issue. Document analysis is a useful preliminary activity for focus group discussions, interviews and observations. Document analysis requires few resources (primarily time to select and analyse the documents), however missing or incomplete documents and limited access to confidential documents are drawbacks.

In the context of PHN intervention management, document analysis includes a review of national, local and organisational mandates for action of relevance to PHN. Reviewing mandates for action is covered in detail in Chapter 9.

Focus group discussions

Forming a focus group is a qualitative research method that brings together participants who share an interest in a certain subject matter and who therefore have particular knowledge or understanding in this subject. It is essentially a group interview process. Focus group participants can be heterogeneous or homogeneous, depending on the purpose of the intelligence-gathering process.[43]

Focus groups can be used to collect information and opinions, to test or get feedback on ideas and suggestions, and to increase the understanding of the different participants on their respective perceptions and approaches. Facilitators direct the discussion process in the group and help to visualise and document arguments and inputs from the participants. Facilitators can support the formulation of action plans if needed and appropriate. Focus groups can make use of tools such as SWOT analysis in order to structure their discussion.

Force field analysis

A force field analysis (FFA) can be used to identify internal and external factors and forces which support or work against the solution of an issue or problem. In the context of formulating a capacity building programme, an FFA may be used to discuss whether suggested capacity building initiatives are feasible or what can be done to make capacity building initiatives possible.[43]

An FFA can present the positive and the negative features of a situation so that they are easily compared with each other. It brings participants to think about different aspects of the desired change and encourages them to agree about the relative priority of factors on each side of the field, thus building consensus for the follow-up activities. The FFA often works best when focusing on the restraining forces rather than the driving forces. It does not require lengthy preparations and infrastructure, but can be applied on the spot as the need arises. Figure 8.2 is a simple example of a force field analysis.

Practice note

Doing a force field analysis and drafting a diagram (as above) is a good exercise to do with key stakeholders as it encourages a dialogue about stakeholder engagement, identifies existing capacity and, most importantly, points to gaps that need attention. It also has a welcome side-effect of increasing stakeholder awareness of the value of working in partnership with other stakeholders.

Force Field
Improvement of nutrition education system for health workers
Ideal state: Training improves individual skills and institutional performance

Driving Factors	*Restraining Factors*
Individual interests in career advancement	Limited funds for training
Improved institutional performance increases standing/ reputation of senior management	Staff placement/career development disconnected from training and skill development
Improved institutional performance leads to increased institutional revenue	Lack of adequate programmes for technical and functional training
Political and public pressure to improve quality of services	Low quality of training
Professional quality assurance system requires staff to accumulate CPD points	Superiors pay little attention to staff skills and competencies
	Existing work culture does not favour introducing changes and innovations

Figure 8.2   Force field analysis
Source: Adapted from GTZ, *Capacity Building Needs Assessment (CBNA) in the Regions (version 2.0)*.[43]

Organisational capacity analysis tools

A number of tools are available (e.g. PROSE and OCAT) to assess and discuss the capacity of an organisation. Many of these have been used in the context of non-public sector organisations; however, they can usually be modified to reflect the specific context of regional government institutions. OCAT differs from PROSE mainly by using an assessment team (i.e. a selection of members from the organisation plus externals) and a variety of data sources for the assessment.

A key element of assessment tools is that it is the organisation's members that assess the capacity of their own organisation. This internal assessment can be complemented by external assessments and by empirical observations/research in order to balance the subjective perception of the members. It is also the members of the organisation who determine the capacity areas and the criteria to be used for each capacity area. This approach ensures that the process of capacity analysis constitutes capacity building, because it engages the members of the organisation in the analysis of the present and the desired condition of their organisation. Both tools create opportunities for two-way learning – a key for institutional capacity building.

Scorecards

A scorecard is a list of characteristics or events against which a Yes/No or numerical score is assigned. These scores are then aggregated and presented as an index. Checklists can effectively track processes, outputs or more general characteristics of an organisation. In addition, they may be used to measure processes or outputs of an organisation correlated to specific areas of capacity development. Scorecards can be used to measure a single capacity component of an organisation or several rolled together. Scorecards/checklists are designed to produce a quantitative score that can be used as an indication of existing capacities or as a target for future capacity building to be achieved. (A scorecard without an aggregate score is also helpful.)

Training needs assessment

One of the most obvious capacity determinants (or resources) in any community is the health workforce. It may also be one of the major gaps in capacity, depending on its level of development. Up-skilling health and community-based professionals in nutrition (workforce development) is one of the most common capacity building strategies used in PHN. This strategy recognises that nutrition guidance and other forms of intervention at the interface with the community can be greatly enhanced in terms of reach and exposure, if primary health carers have access to and apply competencies gained by continuing education and support in nutrition. Needs assessments can provide a mechanism to identify gaps in competency among front-line health workers, in order to focus the capacity building effects of continuing education as a workforce development strategy.

Case study: The Growing Years Project

The Growing Years Project (Gold Coast region, Queensland, Australia) is a multi-strategy, community-based nutrition and physical activity promotion project targeting pregnant women and their infants. A key focus of this project has been around capacity building approaches to intervention management, including assessment of the capacity of the local health workforce to provide effective guidance.

Training needs assessments can use different methods, as illustrated below.

Example 1

The following abstract from a study investigating the education and guidance practices of community-based pharmacists provides an example of how training needs assessment can be conducted.

Mystery shopping

Breastfeeding promotion is universally recognised as a public health imperative with significant impact on health, social and economic outcomes. Among a complex array of determinants that affect breastfeeding initiation and duration, inconsistent advice and support from health professionals is recognised as an unacceptable feature of health service delivery. The role of the community pharmacy as a setting for breastfeeding promotion has received limited attention, despite widespread accessibility, utilisation by women and trust among consumers. In order to assess the quality of guidance practices related to breastfeeding, a pseudo-customer (mystery shopper) study was conducted among a randomly sampled group of 62 pharmacies on the Gold Coast. A mystery shopper (a female dietetic student) was trained to act as the sister of a mother with a seven-week-old baby who was experiencing sore, red and cracked nipples, who was seeking guidance from the pharmacy. Detailed notes of the guidance provided by pharmacy staff were made by the student immediately post-exchange and were compared with observational notes made by a second observer. Analysis of these exchanges indicated almost universal absence (58/62) of pro-active breastfeeding advice and a range of dubious infant formula recommendations that reflect formula company marketing more than the evidence base. This study highlights the need for continuing education for pharmacy staff in infant feeding guidance if the full potential of pharmacy services in this field are to be realised.

Example 2

The following abstract is from a study investigating the continuing education needs of community-based health workers using a self-administered questionnaire.

Needs surveys

Appropriate health education and guidance regarding nutrition and physical activity during key life-stages such as pregnancy and early parenthood are important determinants of healthy behaviours. Primary health care practitioners provide services and guidance at the frontline of the health system. This advice, therefore, needs to be an ongoing focus of service quality considerations. In order to assess the quality of nutrition and physical activity guidance and identify continuing education (CE) needs, this study involved a self-administered survey of primary health practitioners conducted at local health district level. In all 218 surveys were completed capturing a range of primary care system professional groups including medical (n = 58), nursing (n = 55) and community pharmacy (n = 86). The mean (±SD) years' experience of respondents was 14.7 (±11) years. This health workforce sample has regular contact and provides advice to women with infants in the growing years period (one year either side of childbirth) but have varying degrees of confidence regarding the accuracy and currency of their advice. This study has identified gaps in the guidance knowledge base and a range of opportunities and preferences for CE at a local level. These data have been used to develop local health service workforce development strategies as part of the Growing Years Project intervention mix.

Note

Each of these studies has informed the development of a range of localised and specific workforce development strategies including staff up-skilling sessions, nutrition and physical guidance tools and point-of-service education prompts. These studies provide baseline data to support later evaluation of capacity development strategies.

Case study: Capacity assessment checklist

Capacity is often difficult to describe and quantify and has a wide variety of determinants. In an attempt to address this problem and mindful of the need to encourage capacity building practice within PHN practice, a capacity assessment checklist for PHN practice is being developed as a PhD project integrated with the Growing Years Project. The *capacity assessment checklist* (see extract below and appendix 2) attempts to enable rapid assessment of population-level capacity relevant to PHN intervention management. It has been developed from many of the tools and scholarship summarised in this chapter and is intended as a checklist that enables regular assessment (and evaluation) of capacity in the context of interventions. Its aim is to provide directionality to capacity building efforts by using the various capacity determinant modules outlined against the conceptual framework.

This checklist enables a score to be derived for each domain of the Baillie et al.[52] capacity framework (3), which can then be plotted on a spider's web visualisation. Table 8.5 presents one page of the capacity assessment tool, which is also available in the appendix.

Presenting capacity analysis data

Spider's web visualisations are useful if capacity analysis data are in a quantitative form and derived from multiple measurements (e.g. different time-points). Figure 8.3 illustrates how different domains of capacity in the Baillie et al. framework[52] have changed over yearly assessment time-points in the Growing Years Project (not actual data – presented for illustration only).

Table 8.5 Capacity assessment tool – community development domain

COMMUNITY DEVELOPMENT	Contribution to capacity building in community interventions					Evidence
	1 Nil obvious	2 Limited	3 Average	4 Significant	5 Very significant	
Problem identification	There is no obvious identification of the problem by the community	There is limited identification of the issue/problem by the community	There is some identification of the issue by a few sections of the community	There is significant identification of the issue by most sections of the community	There is extensive identification of the issue by a broad representation of the community	
Strategy identification	The community does not obviously identify strategies to deal with the issue	Small sections of the community identify limited strategies to deal with the issue	Some sections of the community identify average strategies to deal with the issue	Many sections of the community identify a significant range of strategies to deal with the issue	A major proportion of the community identify extensive strategies to deal with the issue	
Planning involvement	The community has no obvious involvement in planning interventions to deal with the issue	Small sections of the community have limited involvement in planning interventions to deal with the issue	Some sections of the community have average involvement in planning interventions to deal with the issue	Many sections of the community have significant involvement in planning interventions to deal with the issue	A major proportion of the community has very significant involvement in planning interventions to deal with the issue	
Implementation	The community has no obvious involvement in the implementation of strategies to deal with the issue	Small sections of the community have limited involvement in the implementation of strategies to deal with the issue	Some sections of the community have average involvement in the implementation of strategies to deal with the issue	Many sections of the community have significant involvement in the implementation of strategies to deal with the issue	A major proportion of the community has extensive involvement in the implementation of strategies to deal with the issue	
Service use	The community does not obviously participate in programmes relevant to the issue	Small sections of the community participate in a limited number of programmes relevant to the issue	Some sections of the community participate in an average number of programmes relevant to the issue	Many sections of the community participate in a significant number of programmes relevant to the issue	A major proportion of the community participate extensively in programmes relevant to the issue	
MEAN:						

Source: Libby Baillie & Roger Hughes, University of the Sunshine Coast, Australia for the Growing Years Project, 2008. Used with permission.

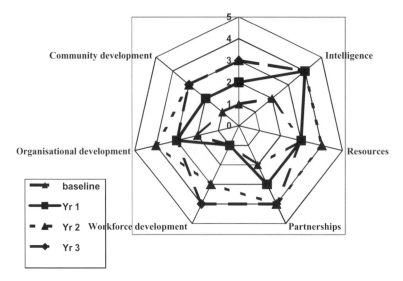

Figure 8.3   Spider's web visualisation of capacity gains over time (from the Growing Years Project)

Key points

- In PHN practice, capacity building relates to the ability and process of individuals, groups, organisations, communities, workforce and systems to perform effective, efficient and sustainable action that achieves objectives such as improved nutrition-related health outcomes.
- Capacity analysis involves identifying and building on existing capacities at each of the various levels (individual, managerial, organisational and systematic) of capacity building, to enable strategy development and establish baseline measures for capacity building evaluation.
- Capacity analysis involves numerous measurement issues and challenges. Selecting tools and strategies that are contextually appropriate and a multi-method process can be used to overcome challenges and enable a comprehensive capacity analysis.
- Strategies to build capacity should be integrated and central to strategy selection and implementation. It is mistaken to assume that strategies can be effective without consideration of how they build capacity and what capacity there is to implement them effectively.
- Establishment of project management committees involving key stakeholders is an important formative capacity building strategy which provides a governance and accountability framework for community intervention management.

Chapter 9

Step 6: Mandates for public health nutrition action

Objectives

On completion of chapter you should be able to:

1. Identify and describe existing local, national and global policy mandates that support PHN intervention management.
2. Describe the importance of understanding the broader policy context when developing PHN interventions.
3. Apply an understanding of policy mandates supporting PHN action in the development of interventions plans and funding proposals.

Practical Public Health Nutrition, first edition. Roger Hughes and Barrie M. Margetts. Published 2011 by Blackwell Publishing Ltd. © 2011 Roger Hughes and Barrie M. Margetts.

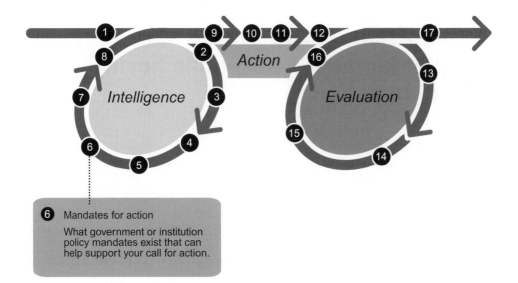

6 Mandates for action

What government or institution policy mandates exist that can help support your call for action.

Introduction

As much of the action required in PHN practice is within the responsibility or jurisdiction of government (public health being a common core function of government in many if not most societies), policy-level commitments are important. Practitioners may consider that policy is beyond an individual professional's practice, however policy exerts a powerful influence on practice because it affects service delivery models and resource allocation and supports or resists actions required to promote public health. It is important, therefore, to gain an understanding of how policies influence the priorities in society that affect the work of PHN. Governments worldwide, with the ever-expanding obesity epidemic adding to the tragic effects of under-nutrition, are developing national nutrition policies and action plans. National nutrition policies set the priorities and strategic direction and provide the framework for PHN action in local communities.

In PHN practice, it is necessary (and strategic) to acknowledge national and organisational mandates in intervention plans and funding submissions. Highlighting how the specific intervention will contribute to prioritised action areas and work plans demonstrates an understanding of the policy context and highlights the intervention's role in supporting the broader public health objectives. Most importantly in this context, alignment of interventions with policy mandates such as action plans makes it easier for government bureaucracies that manage resource distribution for public health action to support your submissions.

Mandates for action – the policy context

The term policy is used in different ways to describe the direction of an organisation or government, a decision to act on a particular problem or a set of guiding principles. The policy context can therefore operate at different levels portraying general values and culture, often used to inform specific targets and action, and/or specific verve on a specified topic.[55] The vast majority of mandates for action which are necessary to review in PHN intervention management are generally considered as policies and include:

- local and national health policies and guidelines;
- national and global policies and guidelines;
- legislation and regulation;
- organisational mission statements and strategic plans;
- professional standards and ethical guidelines.

Public health policy has traditionally related to disease surveillance and control, such as providing a clean water supply, sewage disposal or immunisation. In accordance with contemporary conceptualisations of the environment broadening to include social, cultural and economic aspects (the socio-ecological approach to health), and simple determinant sequences of diseases being replaced with complex causal webs of factors affecting health status, the policy response required is similarly complex,[56] and a vast array of policy areas is considered to have an impact on nutrition-related health problems, including education, food, urban planning, transport, advertising and marketing.

Practice note

Practitioners may consider that policy is beyond an individual professional's practice. However, policy exerts a powerful influence on practice because it affects service delivery models and resource allocation and supports or resists actions required to promote public health. It is important therefore to gain an understanding of how policies influence the priorities in society that affect the work of PHN.[23]

Note that while the policy context is largely considered a top-down process, practitioners are increasingly being invited to contribute to policy development through public consultation, either as individuals or through their organisations and/or professional associations. The outcome of well-evaluated PHN interventions can contribute to the evidence base about effective public health interventions utilised in policy development.

Policy development – an overview

Policy development is a process by which governments or organisations translate their vision into programmes or actions to deliver desired changes. Generally, national governments set the fundamental policy direction, while locally, policies tend to develop incrementally – a series of small steps which do not fundamentally change the status quo.

Policy development follows a basic pathway (similar to programme planning and intervention management), including:

- problem identification and issue recognition;
- policy formulation;
- policy implementation;
- policy evaluation.[57]

This pathway suggests that policy development is a rational process, yet in practice policy-making uses a mix of scientific and pragmatic intelligence. Policy development is also very contextual, subject to the social, cultural, economic and political climate at the time of development.[55]

There are a number of key players involved in policy development, including policy-makers (usually politicians or executive management), policy influences (lobby groups representing vested interests), the public and the media.[23] The level of involvement and role of individual players vary with each issue and are largely dependent on the social climate, the perceived influence of each player, whether players stand to gain or lose from the policy and their ability to have their opinions heard.

Policy development is generally considered the domain of government, typically national government, and in democracies usually follows a sequence of signalling a new policy by circulation of a Green Paper (for public consultation), followed by publication of a White Paper (the government's legislative plan). The policy may proceed through the parliamentary or legislative process to become an Act of Parliament, or may be endorsed by the appropriate Minister or Secretary of State as a statement of intent. (Note that at a global level there is much variation in this policy process, depending on the form of government.

Practice note

Over recent years it has become more common for independent organisations or professional associations to develop policies that publicise their position on particular issues (commonly in the form of a media release) and increase their opportunity to be 'at the table' to bring about improved public health and positive change in government policy. In a recent example several independent organisations, including Which? and the National Heart Forum, were in strong support of an accurate and simplified food labelling scheme. Both organisations have publicised their strong support for the traffic light labelling scheme developed by the Food Standards Agency, and have developed tools to assist consumers use the labels and continue to question government (with various forms of intelligence) about the impact of the scheme in its voluntary form. These health and consumer organisations are considered influential players, along with food manufactures and retailers in this debate.

- Food Standards Agency, *Food Labels: traffic light labelling*, 2008. www.eatwell.gov.uk/foodlabels/trafficlights/
- Which?, *Which? campaigns: Traffic light labelling*, 2008. www.which.co.uk/reports_and_campaigns/food_and_drink/campaigns/nutrition/food_labelling/traffic_light_food_labels_559_116406.jsp
- National Heart Forum, *Nutrition: Traffic-light food labelling*, 2008. www.heartforum.org.uk/Policy_nutrition.aspx?id=4

The challenge of competing policy agendas

For a policy to be developed and adopted, a number of preconditions usually need to be met, including:

- a groundswell of public opinion (social climate);
- a clear definition of the problem;
- concerns voiced by organisations;
- a lack of competing interests or priorities;
- a policy proposal or justified case for the policy;
- support from key political figures who will benefit politically from the policy.

Food and nutrition policies often aspire to ensure the availability and accessibility of healthy foods. Food safety policies ensure protection of health from food contamination. Gaining support for policies that ensure a safe food supply have been popularly and politically supported with the development of national and international policies such as the Codex Alimentaris. However, gaining consensus for policies that encourage the availability and promotion of a healthy food supply is more complex, mostly due to competing and vested interests contributing to the debate. The power and dominance of food manufacturers and retailers compared to that of primary producers and health/consumer organisations, in a climate of globalisation and deregulation, make politicians less likely to introduce regulation or legislation regarding nutrition-related health.

Governments across the world, recently exercised by the global obesity epidemic, are realising their responsibility in addressing population nutrition issues and developing national nutrition policies and action plans. These documents largely aim to protect and promote nutrition-related health and reduce the burden of food-related disease. They therefore represent key policy mandates for PHN action.

National food and nutrition policies

Since the 1992 World Declaration on Nutrition[58] and the resulting Plan of Action on Nutrition and the First Action Plan for Food and Nutrition 2000–2005,[59] there has been considerable effort worldwide (particularly in developed nations such as Australia, New Zealand, Canada and countries in Europe) to develop national policy documents and national plans to address issues directly relevant to PHN. In 2004, a culmination of international political commitment to PHN was observed with the writing of the World Health Organisation (WHO) Global Strategy on Diet, Physical Activity and Health. The objective of the strategy is to provide a basis for concerted action to prevent non-communicable disease.[60] The Global Strategy on Diet, Physical Activity and Health has seen an acceleration of the development and implementation of national policies, plans and programmes to promote lifestyles that include a healthy diet and physical activity.

A review of nutrition policies in the WHO European Region in 2006 found a noticeable improvement in the number of national policy documents focusing on or containing food and nutrition policies, increasing from 24 in 1994 to 45 in 2002.[61] The study showed that 37 countries have final policies, eight have draft documents and three had no nutrition policy documents. Nutrition action areas include infant feeding, food security, food safety, nutrition, physical activity and reducing obesity. Implementation of the policies largely involved establishing advisory groups, food-based dietary guidelines, public nutrition education and monitoring and surveillance systems. Only half of the countries are working inter-sectorally to involve different ministries, the private sector and non-government organisations. The report noted that while many member states have developed policies related to food and nutrition, implementation still appears to be a major challenge. Specific implementation challenges include lack of funds, political commitment, coordination and/or expertise.

Practice note

It is important to recognise that national action plans, as instruments of government/politics, are not perfect and often represent modest intent rather than action. For example, most still focus on 'informed choice and individual responsibility' as the primary model and they usually avoid confronting industry and/or using fiscal policies to drive change. Rarely do they commit further funding and it is often unclear how the actions outlined will be implemented. Nonetheless, they are important drivers of resource allocation decision-making relevant to practitioners wanting to develop interventions.

Mandates for action – direct relevance to PHN practice

The impact and relevance of nutrition policies and action plans in the context of PHN practice are significant. National nutrition policies and action plans articulate a commitment by government and other signatories or partners to the public health of citizens and provide a national government-level mandate for action on population nutrition issues. Referring to and aligning action to these policies and action plans can be very important in terms of influencing regional and local resource allocation to issues such as workforce development, intervention funding and development.

National nutrition policies and action plans codify national government priorities for action. By highlighting the nutrition areas for action and target groups the PHN workforce effort can be focused and be more effective at achieving the desired health outcomes. Implementation of the strategic priorities outlined in national nutrition policies and action plans requires a workforce that can build the capacity of communities to effectively design, plan, implement and evaluate strategies that are sustainable. Hence, both national nutrition policies and PHN intervention management are required to solve population nutrition problems. National nutrition policies set the strategic direction and (usually) provide the framework and resources for PHN action in local communities. Successful local action relies on public health nutritionists taking a bottom-up approach, building community capacity for sustainable change and feeding evaluation results back to policy-makers through literature publications and consultation contributions.

Practice note

Being aware of the budget allocation attached to national nutrition policies and action plans, and the various strategies within, is vital when trying to secure funding for local activities. It is important to note that many national mandates for action involve a collaboration of ministries, which means that funding opportunities may come from the Department of Education, Agriculture, Community Services or Planning and not exclusively from the Department for Health. Noting annual government budget announcements is also essential in order to be aware of potential pools of money which may be applied for to support PHN interventions.

In any application, be sure to link your planned intervention to the strategic direction and actions outlined in the national nutrition policy. Where possible, make explicit reference to how your intervention plan addresses priorities and strategic directions outlined in national action plans.

National nutrition policies and action plans are not the only mandates for action that need to be considered in PHN intervention management. It is also necessary to consider the mandates of your own organisation, potential partners or competitors and possible funding agencies. Other mandates for action that may require review, depending on the type of intervention, include relevant legislation and regulation, policies and guidelines or professional and ethical standards.

The importance of reviewing the mandate for action or strategic plan of your own organisation and partnering organisations is to ensure managerial and executive support of the proposed intervention. Presenting the intervention as a contribution to the focused action for the organisation will help gain managerial support, while identifying commonalities will strengthen intervention partnerships.

Reviewing the strategic plans of competing organisations enhances awareness of their key objectives and can assist with developing strategies to deal with potential objections to the proposed intervention. A vast number of organisations make their strategic plans available on their website or in their annual report; they are also usually available on request.

Aligning intervention objectives with the key strategic directions of a potential funding agency is essential to secure any financial assistance. There are many potential funding agencies and the topic, nature and design of the particular PHN intervention will assist in determining which funding agency is most likely to provide financial support to your particular intervention. Local projects are commonly supported by local or regional agencies (health boards, local municipalities) or funding grants from commercial agencies with a philanthropic arm (e.g. health insurance companies, etc.). Broader funding opportunities may be available from the European Union or European Commission. Currently, the Public Health Programme 2008–2013 provides funding to health interventions across member countries. When making submissions to a funding agency it is vital to make clear how the intended PHN intervention contributes to the agency's action plan and that the intervention is strategically relevant (i.e. tied to national, regional government nutrition policies). The Public Health Programme, for example, has three overarching health objectives plus annual work plan priority areas. Applicants must spell out in their application how the intervention contributes to these priority areas and outline the intervention's strategic relevance to European and national policy direction.

Practice note

Funding agencies and government bodies want to see that the interventions they are financing contribute to the prioritised health objectives. Knowing the national and organisational mandates for action is a vital component of PHN intervention management and must be addressed in intervention plans and funding submissions. Highlighting how your intervention will contribute to priority action areas and work plans demonstrates your understanding of the policy context and your interventions role in supporting the broader public health objectives. In short, this makes it easier for bureaucrats to support your plans.

Key points

- National nutrition policies and action plans codify national government priorities for action. By highlighting the nutrition areas for action and target groups, the PHN workforce effort can be focused and be more effective at achieving the desired health outcomes.
- National nutrition policies and PHN intervention management are both required in solving population nutrition problems. National nutrition policies set the strategic direction and provide the framework for PHN action in local communities. PHN interventions build community capacity for sustainable change. Intervention evaluation results in feedback to policy-makers through literature publications and consultation.
- Considering the existing mandates of your own organisation, potential partners or competitors and possible funding agencies is necessary in PHN interventions to gain managerial and executive support and strengthen intervention partnerships.
- Linking the national and organisational mandates to PHN interventions must be addressed in intervention plans and funding submissions. Highlighting how the intervention will contribute to priority action areas and work plans demonstrates an understanding of the policy context and the intervention's role in supporting the broader public health objectives.

Chapter 10

Step 7: Intervention research and strategy options

Objectives

On completion of this chapter you should be able to:

1. Apply health promotion strategic frameworks to identify strategic approaches to address the determinants of PHN problems.
2. Identify and analyse intelligence from prior PHN and broader intervention research and evaluation to inform intervention design and strategy selection.
3. Identify and justify strategy options to assist intervention design decision-making.

Practical Public Health Nutrition, first edition. Roger Hughes and Barrie M. Margetts. Published 2011 by Blackwell Publishing Ltd. © 2011 Roger Hughes and Barrie M. Margetts.

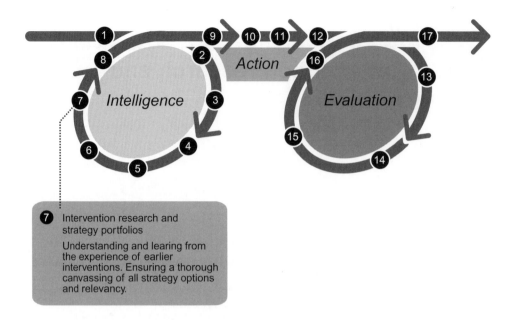

7 Intervention research and strategy portfolios

Understanding and learing from the experience of earlier interventions. Ensuring a thorough canvassing of all strategy options and relevancy.

Introduction

By this stage (step 7) in the practice bi-cycle you should have a good understanding of the problem, its causes and which determinants are priorities for intervention (if not, further investigation of the issue may be required before a solution can be developed). The next task is to decide what strategies can be applied to best address the determinants of the issue. PHN interventions are usually made up of a mix of strategies – strategies being purposely designed activities that work to change determinants of a PHN problem. It is important to know how others have addressed similar issues, the strategy mix they used, the sequence of strategies, key lessons from others' efforts and how all this can be used to fine-tune the strategies to be used for your situation. You don't want to reinvent the wheel, but rather improve it! These are the questions that inspire intervention research. A conceptual understanding of the different strategy options, levels of action, settings and target groups is a prerequisite for critical intervention research and strategy prioritisation. Intervention research is an intelligence-gathering process that helps with decision-making in the intervention design process.

Strategic frameworks for health promotion

Table 10.1, based on UK-based Nuffield Foundation's intervention ladder, suggests that there is a continuum of strategy approaches which vary in terms of the extent to which

Table 10.1   The public health intervention ladder

	Strategy	Example
Increasingly unpopular yet effective strategy	Eliminate choice	Ban junk foods
	Restrict choice	Remove trans-saturated fat from manufactured foods
	Guide choice through disincentives	Tax fatty foods
	Guide choice through incentives	Subsidise fresh fruit and vegetables so they are low cost
	Guide choice through changing default policy	Salad as a side-dish instead of chips
	Enable choice	Increase the availability of fruit and vegetables relative to junk food
	Provide information	Television advertising promoting fruit and vegetable consumption
	Do nothing or monitor situation	

Source: Adapted from nuffieldbioethics.org.

they consider individual choice and public health as priorities. These are often contradictory and a point of considerable debate – for example, to what extent should individuals have the freedom to participate in risky health-related behaviours such as smoking, high-fat food consumption, alcohol abuse, etc.? vs. the responsibility of the state to limit choices in the public interest.

There are a number of strategic frameworks developed through the World Health Organisation and the health promotion community that are useful when considering the types of strategies to employ in PHN interventions. These frameworks highlight the importance of delivering interventions with a mix of strategies across a range of action areas. The Ottawa Charter for Health Promotion[16] was developed at the first International Conference on Health Promotion in 1986, and the five key action areas proposed there have been widely used. They continue to have currency in practice after more than two decades and are considered central to effective health promotion practice. Statements from International Health Promotion conferences since Ottawa (Adelaide 1988, Sunsvall 1991, Jakarta 1997, Mexico 2000, Bangkok 2005, Vancouver 2007) have added to the strategic frameworks applicable to PHN practice (summarised in Table 10.2).

Table 10.2   Strategy options: action areas for health promotion

Action		Application in public health nutrition practice	Example
OTTAWA CHARTER (3)	Building healthy public policy *Regulate and legislate to ensure a high level of protection from harm and enable equal opportunity for health wellbeing for all people*	Involves putting nutrition and health on the agenda of policy-makers in all sectors and at all levels (national/local government, childcare, schools, workplaces, food industry), directing them to be aware of the health consequences of their decisions and accept their responsibilities for health.	Legislation, fiscal measures, taxation and organisational change that promotes better nutrition.
	Creating supportive environments	The inextricable link between people and their environment constitutes the basis for a socio-ecological approach to health. Work and leisure should be a source of health for people. We have a responsibility to take care of each other, our communities and our national environment. Health promotion generates living and working conditions that are safe, stimulating, satisfying and enjoyable.	*The availability and accessibility of fruit and vegetables in schools, workplaces and communities is an important environmental factor relevant to nutritional health.*

Table 10.2 *Continued*

Action		Application in public health nutrition practice	Example
	Strengthening community action	Health promotion works through concrete and effective community action in setting priorities, making decisions, planning strategies and become the core implementers to achieve better health.	*At the heart of this process is the empowerment of communities – community ownership and control over determining the nutrition-related health issues of importance to them.*
	Developing personal skills	Health promotion supports personal and social development through providing information, education for health and enhancing life skills. Information, education and skills can increase the options available to people to exert more control over their own health and their environments.	*Producing, selecting, preparing and consuming foods that promote good health depend on knowledge and skills.*
	Reorienting health services	Health services need to embrace an expanded mandate that supports the needs of individuals and communities for a healthier life, and opens channels between the health sector and broader social, political, economic and physical environmental components.	*Community dietitians reducing the hours they spend in outpatient clinics for weight reduction and instead working with the community to implement community-based strategies to address overweight issue is an example of health service reorientation.*
JAKARTA DECLARATION	Promote social responsibility for health	Decision-makers must be firmly committed to social responsibility. Both the public and private sectors should promote health by pursuing policies and practices that do not harm individual health, protect the environment, restrict production of and trade in inherently harmful goods, safeguard citizens in the marketplace and workplace, and include equity-focused health impact assessments in policy development.	*Legislation that requires food manufacturers to list ingredients, nutrient profiles and specific warnings to assist consumer choice and promote transparency.*

Table 10.2 *Continued*

Action	Application in public health nutrition practice	Example
Increase investments for health development	Current investment in health is commonly inadequate and ineffective. Increasing investment for development requires a multi-sectoral approach, where investments reflect the needs of particular groups such as indigenous, older people and marginalised populations.	*Investment in PHN workforce development among indigenous populations building capacity for community self-help.*
Consolidate and expand partnerships for health *Partner and build alliances with public, private, NGOs and civil society to create sustainable actions*	Health promotion requires partnership across sectors and at all levels of governance and society. Partnerships should offer mutual benefit for health by sharing expertise, skills and resources, and be based on respect, agreed ethical principles and transparency.	*Developing partnerships between health services, universities, schools and community organisations to promote nutrition in the school setting. Each member brings resources to the partnership to enhance capacity for effective action.*
Increase community capacity and empower the individual *Build capacity for policy development, leadership, health promotion practice, knowledge transfer and research, and health literacy*	Health promotion is carried out by and with people, not on or to people. It improves the capacity of both the individual and society to take action and influence the determinants of health. Building community capacity requires practical education to build health literacy, leadership training and access to intelligence from research and resources.	*Involving community members in defining needs and selecting strategy priorities, building and supporting leadership within communities and sharing intelligence from research to inform community decision-making.*

Text in italics = Bangkok Declaration adaptations.[64]

The Jakarta Declaration on Leading Health Promotion into the 21st Century[62] was developed at the fourth International Conference on Health Promotion in 1997. It builds on the Ottawa Charter and further endorses the need for comprehensive approaches, family and community participation, and across-sector partnerships (including with the private sector). The Jakarta Declaration clearly confirms the importance of considering capacity building strategies and securing adequate social resources, infrastructure and responsibility when implementing health promotion interventions.[63] The Bangkok Charter for Health Promotion (2005)[64] emphasised the critical importance of advocacy for health, capacity building (again) and the important role of government in regulating and legislating to protect the public.

Determinants as leverage points for intervention

In step 4 of the PHN intervention management bi-cycle (determinant analysis), determinants were identified. Determinants represent the factors that need to be changed in order to facilitate improvements in the problem being addressed. They therefore represent intervention leverage points that can help focus strategy selection. Note that determinants can be modifiable (e.g. knowledge) and non-modifiable (e.g. gender), so prioritisation needs to focus on determinants that feasibly can be changed. Table 10.3 summarises determinants of food choice as leverage points for population-based nutrition interventions. The determinants of food choice are classified against the ecological model of health and as either modifiable or non-modifiable.

Levels of intervention

The socio-ecological approach to public health recognises that there are numerous levels of influence in populations, which means that PHN interventions must be directed appropriately at the level of greatest impact.

Table 10.4 presents three levels at which PHN interventions can focus and provides examples of interventions at each of these levels. It is important to note that all three levels are usually required for a comprehensive approach to a PHN problem and that the best mix of interventions depends on the situation and the resources available.

Settings as a focus for intervention

Settings refer to physical environments in which people live, access services, work and play. Settings offer opportunities for comprehensive interventions which can be directed at health behaviour change and environmental change to achieve improved health outcomes. Settings also offer an opportunity to reach specific target populations, such as mothers through child and maternal health clinics and teenagers through schools. Successful health promotion through different settings will be characterised by comprehensive interventions achieving change in both behavioural and environmental determinants of health.

Table 10.3 Determinants of food choice as leverage points for intervention in PHN practice

	Determinant	Modifiable?
Intra-personal		
Biological	Gender	No
	Age	No
	Race/ethnicity	No
Psychological	Self-efficacy	Yes
	Expectations	Yes
	Values	Yes
	Perceived norms	Yes
	Perceived barriers	Yes
	Stress	Yes
Behavioural	Food-related skills	Yes
	Dietary behaviours	Yes
	Physical activity behaviours	Yes
	TV viewing	Yes
	Transportation choices	Yes
Socio-environmental		
Social community	Mass-media programmes	Yes
	Community nutrition programmes	Yes
	Culturally-based food practices	Yes
	Neighbourhood socioeconomic status	Yes
	Workplace environment and policies	Yes
Demographic	Employment	Yes
	Income	Yes
	Education	Yes
Physical environment		
Community	Food availability	Yes
	Food prices	Yes
	Point-of-sale food promotions	Yes
	Food accessibility	Yes
Demographic	Household structure	?
Policy context		
Policy	Food related policies and programmes	Yes
	Transport policies	Yes

Source: Adapted from French.[65]

Settings of relevance to PHN practice

- Maternal and/or childcare, community centres.
- Elders' clubs.
- Communities, such as defined population groups (a village, a suburb).
- Food service – takeaways, restaurants, caterers.
- Food supply – retailers, manufacturers, producers.
- Health institutions – hospitals, nursing homes.
- Schools/educational institutions.
- Workplaces.

Table 10.4   Levels of intervention as a focus for PHN intervention design

Levels of population based intervention	Description	Example from public health nutrition practice
Community-focused practice *Social/cultural*	Community-focused practice changes community norms, community attitudes and community behaviours. Directed at entire communities and measured in terms of what proportion of the population changes.	Use of social marketing strategies (e.g. posters, advertising, etc.) to challenge negative community attitudes e.g. about breastfeeding in public or weekly iron and folic acid supplementation to reduce anaemia in young women before they get married.
Systems-focused practice *Policy/ environmental*	Interventions at this level change environments, organisations, policies, laws and power structures. The focus is on systems that affect health. Changing systems is often more effective and long-lasting than individual change approaches.	Changing the nutritional composition of takeaway food by training retailers in best practice chip cooking methods; manufacturers reduce salt, fat and/or sugar content of processed foods.
Individual-focused practice *Intrapersonal*	Changes knowledge, attitudes, beliefs, practices and behaviours of individuals. This practice level is directed at risk-identified individuals and social networks (e.g. families or other community groups).	Increasing the skills of community members in food budgeting to address food insecurity among low-income groups (if this is key constraint).

Source: Adapted from Keller et al.[66]

Target groups as a focus for intervention

A focus on particular population or target groups allows for better targeting of health problems which are more common among that particular group; it may facilitate greater participation in interventions in that group.

Addressing health problems among disadvantaged populations may also encourage interventions that address the underlying social, cultural, economic and political determinants of health, such as poverty, culture and employment status, access to resources and services, and which can assist in reducing health inequalities. To address a health problem in a particular population (the primary target population), interventions may need to be achieved through a different target group (the secondary target population).

For example, childhood obesity may require engaging and working with parents and carers, childcare centre staff and local government decision-makers rather than working specifically with the children of the community.

The success of an intervention may be defined in terms of the opportunities for community participation and the ability to achieve change in the structural determinants of health or behaviour.

Intervention research: learning from earlier work

Intervention research is an important source of intelligence about the features of earlier intervention successes and failures. Researching previous and current interventions serves to identify what does and doesn't work, when, to what extent and under what circumstances. Details about the various strategy options that may be used or modified to the context of your particular scenario can be identified, listed and appraised systematically to reveal an appropriate strategy mix for your intervention.

Intervention research is interested in answering the following questions:

- What strategies can be applied to address the determinants of the identified population nutrition issue?
- How have others addressed a similar issue? What strategy mix and sequence of strategies were used?
- What was the logic applied in strategy selection? Was there a clear link between the problem analysis and strategy intent?
- What change did their intervention demonstrate?
- What resource investment was required to achieve their intervention results?
- What challenges were others presented with? How can their lessons be used to improve the strategy implementation in your intervention?

Intervention research focuses on taking an intelligence-based approach to PHN practice by using evidence from health promotion research and programme evaluation. Strong evidence of intervention and strategy *efficacy* can be found in systematic reviews, where the evidence is commonly derived from experimental or quasi-experimental studies. However, there are very few randomised control trials that evaluate public health nutrition intervention *effectiveness*, largely because the key strategies of participation, community empowerment, policy development and environmental change present a greater challenge for robust evaluation than individually oriented behaviour change.[16] It has also been noted that there is commonly a mismatch between the types of interventions that have been rigorously evaluated and those used in community-based practice, which further limits the depth of the evidence base available to practitioners.[67]

It is important to use a variety of intelligence sources when conducting intervention research. Three principal forms of intelligence include:

1   *Published literature* – Published intervention research can provide strategy utilisation and evaluation insights, particularly for common intervention settings such as schools and childcare centres. However, finding PHN community-based evaluation

evidence can be difficult because of the limited capacity to publish intervention research. Literature reviews on other health promotion issues with intervention success, such as smoking, can be a useful prompt for innovation and new approaches. Databases such as the Cochrane Collaboration and NHS Centre for Reviews and Dissemination may be useful.

2 *Grey literature* – The development of the web has increased access to non-peer reviewed reports. These can be a rich source of PHN intervention research intelligence. Try surfing the net or searching the websites (e.g. www.cdc.gov).

3 *Professional networks and 'practice wisdom'* – Using professional networks to scan for information about strategy options is also recommended. Colleagues are likely to have tried different strategies and have experience and unpublished intelligence that may be relevant to your situation. Contacting colleagues by telephone, emailing questions through list-serves or contacting university-based colleagues with intelligence from student projects or their own research are all useful ways of adding intelligence to your intervention research. It is important to note that your intervention evaluation will contribute to the PHN intelligence pool and will be an important source of intelligence for future intervention planning so keep records of lessons learnt, etc.

Practice note

When conducting intervention research it is useful to start by searching for systematic reviews on your particular issue or problem. Try the Cochrane collection at www.cochrane.org. Systematic reviews can be limited in the area of public health nutrition so it is also valuable to conduct keyword searches (based on your identified determinants) in databases such as PubMed and Medline. It is also worth considering searching in databases of relevance to your determinants outside the health sector. Urban planning, transport, the food industry or marketing can provide useful examples of interventions that are addressing the determinants that also affect health. Remember also to conduct a keyword search in the web to find unpublished literature and to phone or email colleagues about interventions they have tried or are aware of. All this intelligence will help identify a range of strategy options for your intervention.

Librarians can be an important resource as they are specialists in sourcing information.

Abstracting intelligence from intervention research

Using a systematic approach to reviewing and organising intelligence from the literature is an important practice discipline and can greatly assist critical review of strategy options for intervention design. An abstraction table is presented in Table 10.5. The focus of intervention research as a prelude to intervention design should focus on the following questions:

• Which determinants did strategies address?
• How have others addressed similar situations and with what strategy mix/sequence of strategies?

Table 10.5   Abstraction table

Reference details	Description of problem addressed	Strategy mix description	Evidence of effect	Evaluation method	Lessons/ intelligence gain
Example only: Simpson, H., I've only got money for fries. *Springfield J Pub Hlth*, 2005	High intake of fatty, takeaway food among middle-aged obese men working in a power plant, contributing to high percentage on sick leave	Project involved men in a cooking competition, which included skill development in cooking, purchasing and presentation of food	Sick leave reduced after 12 months. Proportion of men obese reduced by 10% over 12 months. Fatty, takeaway food consumption decreased	Pre- and post-intervention analysis of sick leave records, three-day diet histories and physical screenings	Men participate in health promotion activities if a competition is involved. Up-skilling successfully addressed major determinant of food preparation incompetence.
Etc.					

- What was the logic applied in strategy selection? Was there a clear link between what the strategies were trying to achieve and the analysis of the problem?
- What sort of change did other interventions demonstrate?
- What sort of resource investment was required to achieve these results?
- What lessons (intelligence) can be gleaned from others' efforts, and how can this be used to fine-tune the strategies used for your situation?

Key points

- An understanding of the different strategy options and levels of action are prerequisites for critical intervention research. Strategies are the activities undertaken as part of the intervention to resolve the health issue. A number of well-developed and effective strategies can be used in a multi-strategy PHN intervention. In determining what comprehensive action to take on a population nutrition issue, the full range of intervention types needs to be considered.
- Intervention research is an important source of intelligence about the features of health promotion intervention success. Researching previous and current interventions serves to help identify what works, when and in what circumstances and focuses the strategy options available for use or modified to your PHN situation.
- It is important to use a variety of intelligence sources when conducting intervention research. The three principal forms of intelligence are: published literature, grey literature and professional networks.
- Presenting intervention research results by compiling tables of strategies, their settings and target group against each of the determinants of the identified issue can provide a good basis for discussion of the range of possible interventions to address the identified population nutrition issue.

Useful websites

Strategy frameworks for health promotion

- World Health Organisation/Canadian Public Health Association/Health and Welfare Canada, *Ottawa Charter for Health Promotion*, 1986. First International Conference on Health Promotion: Ottawa. Visit. www.who.int/hpr/NPH/docs/ottawa_charter_hp.pdf.
- World Health Organisation, *The Jakarta Declaration on Leading Health Promotion into the 21st Century*, 1997. Fourth International Conference on Health Promotion: Jakarta. www.who.int/hpr/NPH/docs/jakarta_declaration_en.pdf.

Intervention research

- The Cochrane Collaboration, www.cochrane.org.
- Review of health promotion and education online, rhpeo.org.
- NHS Centre for Reviews and Dissemination, www.york.ac.uk/inst/crd.
- Centre for Disease Control and Prevention, www.cdc.gov.

Strategy abstraction examples

- Gill, T., King, L. & Webb, K., Best options for promoting healthy weight and preventing weight gain in NSW, 2005, www.cphn.mmb.usyd.edu.au.

Chapter 11

Step 8: Risk assessment and strategy prioritisation

Objectives

On completion of this chapter you should be able to:

1. Apply risk management concepts and processes to predict and manage potential positive and negative effects of public health nutrition interventions.
2. Understand and explain the importance of risk identification and management in PHN intervention management.
3. Apply transparent decision-making processes to aid prioritisation of strategies when designing PHN interventions.
4. Identify key dilemmas and challenges of strategy prioritisation.

Practical Public Health Nutrition, first edition. Roger Hughes and Barrie M. Margetts. Published 2011 by Blackwell Publishing Ltd. © 2011 Roger Hughes and Barrie M. Margetts.

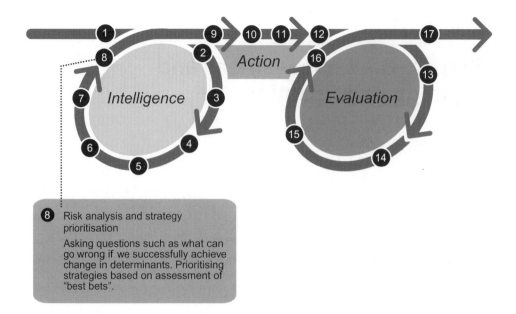

8 Risk analysis and strategy prioritisation

Asking questions such as what can go wrong if we successfully achieve change in determinants. Prioritising strategies based on assessment of "best bets".

Introduction

Before progressing to the action stage of intervention management, consideration of the risks associated with action (and/or inaction) is a professional and ethical responsibility in practice. In health care the maxim 'first do no harm' applies as much to prevention approaches as it does to clinical intervention. Risk assessment (the initial phase of a process of managing risk) focuses on considering the risks associated with doing nothing and then the risks associated with the implementation of strategies. Sometimes, the best intentions can create other problems that may be greater than those we originally set out to address. Risk assessment enables practitioners to foresee and plan to manage risks as well as clearly identify the anticipated benefits of intervention. If the risks outweigh the benefits, there is no good reason to persist with an intervention in its current form.

A key challenge in PHN intervention management is to prioritise and select the best mix of strategies to address modifiable determinants effectively, within context and mindful of the existing capacity to implement sustainably. Selecting and prioritising intervention strategies appropriately involves analysing the risks and benefits associated with these determinants.

Assessing risks and benefits

Decisions about whether a determinant (identified in the earlier analytical stage of the practice framework) becomes a focus of a PHN intervention and should be a function of the measurable or estimated risk or benefit associated with that determinant.[68] While risk and benefit assessment does not represent all the considerations relevant to action on a determinant, it does provide a valuable source of information to be used in strategy prioritisation.

Risk refers to the probability that a hazard will result in an adverse health event.
Benefit refers to the probability that a protective/promotive factor will result in a positive health event.

The decision whether to take action or not depends on:

- the prevalence of the problem/issue;
- the evidence linking the determinant to the health issue;
- the actual or potential size of the impact on health – both the risks and the benefits;
- the effectiveness of the action and capacity to intervene and are addressed in more detail through the process of strategy prioritisation.

An assessment of the risks and benefits associated with determinants provides information to assist in deciding whether a determinant should be managed and to prioritise among determinants and will be of assistance later in strategy prioritisation. Risks and benefits are revealed by considering the nature, likelihood and severity of adverse effects and positive factors on health.[68]

The assessment process needs to consider a number of key issues:

- the likelihood of the health risk or benefit;
- which individuals and groups are most at risk or will derive most benefit;
- the severity of the anticipated adverse impacts or the size of the expected benefit;
- the potential to prevent the effects or to succeed in providing the benefits;
- the nature and strength of evidence which supports the conclusion about the nature and magnitude of the risk or benefit;
- the range of informed views and confidence about the evidence;
- other sources causing the same type of risk;
- the distribution of the risk or potential benefit in relation to other risks and benefits in the population;
- the impacts other than those on health (e.g. social or cultural consequences).[48]

Stakeholders play an important role in providing information for use in risk and benefit assessment, reinforcing the need for ongoing stakeholder engagement outlined in earlier stages of the intervention cycle. Most stakeholders will identify specific concerns which are of relevance to them, such that perceptions can vary substantially among stakeholders and assessment may be highly controversial, especially when information is lacking. The decision to take action, to manage risks and promote benefits should be based on scientific assessment. However, decisions to act must be taken even if information about the potential risks is lacking or incomplete. Managing risks and benefits should reflect a preference for avoiding unnecessary health risks rather than unnecessary expenditure.[68]

Case study: Risk and benefit assessment – increasing fruit and vegetable intake

Research has shown that eating more fruit and vegetables may be the single most important dietary change needed to reduce the risk of major chronic diseases, while the risk of adverse effects of increasing fruit and vegetable consumption appears to be small. Increasing fruit and vegetable intake to the recommended levels will displace other less nutrient-dense and energy-rich foods from the diet and increase exposure to dietary components that reduce disease risk. Levels of pesticide residues and other contaminants (*a potential and perceived risk*) remain well below threshold levels at recommended intake levels. The economic costs to consumers is a concern in some sectors (*a potential barrier and/or risk*); however, assessments have shown that consuming more plant-based foods and less energy-dense foods reduces total food costs. Increasing population consumption of fruit and vegetables is likely to require increased and improved production and handling of fruit and vegetables, which will have some technological, economic and social impacts, and estimates of potential impact on the fruit and vegetable industry should be undertaken.[48]

The importance of context

In India in the rainy season, faecal contamination of green leafy vegetables can be a problem, and women there have told us that they don't eat them because they get diarrhoea and so see no benefit. This reinforces the need to explore and consider issues in consultation with key stakeholders.

Types of risks and benefits

There are three types of risks and benefits to health to be considered:

1 *Expressed* – a risk or benefit has a consistent link between the determinant and health issue, and can be measured.
2 *Potential* – a risk or benefit that relates to a sporadic, unreported or non-existent health issue such that the prevalence of the determinant can only be estimated.
3 *Perceived* – a risk or benefit that occurs when there is strong public perception that intervention is desirable despite the lack of scientific evidence to support action.[68]

All three types require consideration and attention in the risk analysis and strategy prioritisation process.

Practice note

In practice, people in a community that you engage with may not *perceive* the risk associated with poor nutrition. The community may instead identify immediate issues such as drug abuse, HIV or other infectious diseases as the primary risks they are concerned about rather than *expressed risk* such as inadequate fruit and vegetable intake (contributing to increased risk of certain cancers, cardiovascular disease, etc.) even though the expressed risk may have a greater impact on health. Exploring differences between expressed, perceived and potential risks is important because it may influence the strategies required to ensure ongoing community participation.

Strategy prioritisation

In practice, intervention design is a compromise between the best possible strategy mix given unlimited resources and the reality of limited resources and associated capacity. Strategy prioritisation is the task of ranking and ordering identified strategies to assist with the development of a strategy portfolio. The word *portfolio* in this sense is used in much the same way that financial market investors will buy shares on the stock market, after weighing up the risks and benefits (in this case whether stocks will increase or decrease in value) and deciding on the mix of shares to invest in. Resources for PHN interventions are commonly limited (sometimes very limited) and deciding which strategies to use and which to reject can be difficult. Hence, strategy portfolio selection involves practitioners prioritising strategies to identify and select the *best buys* (i.e. the strategies most likely to solve the PHN problem and contribute to health improvements, relative to cost/investment).

Strategy prioritisation is best developed through a collaborative decision-making process, where key stakeholders consider all the available intelligence on the health problem and the known strategy options/interventions to address the problem.[68] Using criteria with specific definitions can help to standardise and make more objective what is typically a largely subjective process.[69] The choice and definition of each criterion component, and relative weighting scheme, should be based on group consensus, typically agreed by the project team or project management committee, and open to critical analysis and scrutiny by the public/target group and decision-makers.[68] Allowing public scrutiny and debate of the criteria illustrates transparency of the priority setting and decision-making and helps convince non-specialists that the process is not biased or risky. It also assists with the empowerment of the community (see the Growing Years Project case study below as an example).

Challenges and dilemmas in strategy prioritisation

Agreeing on priorities and selecting strategies for an intervention is a complex task that requires practitioners to use their negotiation and collaboration skills. The process of strategy prioritisation and selection is complicated by the:

- *Vast range of strategy possibilities* – There are many possible strategies that could be implemented to address a PHN problem, as identified through the intervention research (step 7). Prioritising these strategies in a systematic, transparent manner can be challenging, particularly when several stakeholders are involved.[69] A number of tools are available to assist with analysis of all the information on the problem and situation such that the strategy can be considered in context and prioritised accordingly. Potentially useful approaches/tools, including the Angelo Framework[70] and ACE process,[71] are discussed in more detail below.
- *Level of evidence available for prevention strategies* – Ideally, strategy prioritisation should be based on the highest level of evidence, preferably a systematic review of scientific studies that demonstrate a strong link between the strategy and the desired outcome. It is important to recognise, however, that this level of evidence may be difficult to achieve in all cases and should not prevent action from being taken if the evidence points in one direction and plausible alternative explanations are not present.

Practice note

One of the real gaps in the intelligence base that limits intervention design decision-making is a lack of evidence about intervention effectiveness. This is due to a number of factors, including limited evaluation practice and difficulty in evaluating population-based intervention effects. PHN interventions are trying to solve complex problems in complex communities and involve complex strategy portfolios. This complexity makes PHN interventions difficult to evaluate in well-controlled evaluation studies.

- *Resource limitations* – PHN interventions are commonly restricted by resource limitations, including limited funding, staff capacity and equipment for adequate implementation of identified strategies. Strategy prioritisation needs to match the implementation capacity.[72] Results from the capacity analysis (step 6) will assist in identifying and prioritising within the contextual capacity limitations.

Methods for strategy prioritisation

The priority rating process: one method to help prioritise interventions

The prioritisation model developed by Pickett and Hanlon[69] is useful for comparing different and competing strategies to address determinants of a health problem and to identify the key considerations in strategy prioritization. The model incorporates factors of health problem or determinant, including the *size, seriousness, effectiveness* and *contextual appropriateness* of available strategies, to numerically prioritise health needs and interventions.[73]

Using the intelligence and data gathered from the earlier steps of the intervention management bi-cycle, the analysis team work to determine agreed definitions of each of the four components of the model. Each component is scored and then applied to the following formula and then the basic priority rating (BPR) is calculated.

$$BPR = [(A+B) \times C/3] \times D$$

The four components of the model are:

1 *Size of the problem (A)* – total score: 0–10
   The size of the problem is scored by the number of individuals in a population at risk of, or suffering from, the problem.
   Example scoring scale: *Number score*
   50 000 + 10
   5000 – 49 999 8
   500 – 4999 6
   50 – 499 4
   5 – 49 2
   0.5 – 4.9 0

2 *Seriousness of the problem (B)* – total score: 0–20
   Defined in terms in four factors:

   – *Urgency* – the nature of the problem and sense of community urgency.

   – *Severity* – based on the fatality rate estimates or seriousness of the disability.

   – *Economic loss* – this may reflect community and family/individual losses.

   – *Involvement of others* – most commonly this relates to health problems that are highly contagious.

3 *Effectiveness of strategies (C)* – total score: 0–10
   Most groups can make reasonably useful estimates based on previous evaluation or research results. For example, if a strategy reaches only 20% of the population and is only 70% effective, then the statistical score is 14% – a low rating. Effectiveness is a multiplier in the formula and therefore has a powerful impact.

4 *PEARL – propriety, economics, acceptability, resources, legality (D)* – total score: 0 or 1

PEARL determines whether an intervention can be carried out given that the basic priority rating is a product of the product of a score of either 0 or 1. The score is allocated by considering each element as possible or not. For example, are there adequate or inadequate resources to implement the strategy?

The analysis team need to work together to determine the BPR for each strategy using a consistent definition and scoring system for each of the four components. The process will be unique to the situation and should be consistent and transparent.[69]

The priority rating process approach to strategy prioritisation was developed for traditional public health problems and has several limitations when applied to PHN primary prevention intervention management, including:

• There is limited evidence of intervention effectiveness for many PHN strategies.
• Change/effectiveness of PHN strategies is relatively small.
• Measurements of PHN strategies is of limited quality effectiveness.

Practice note

The mathematical process described above may seem very analytical and pedantic. However, its application in PHN practice can help identify the different considerations required when prioritising the focus of intervention design.

The next case study illustrates the process that can be used to engage stakeholders in collaborative strategy prioritisation, using a range of assessment criteria and focusing on identifying strategy 'best buys'. This process was conducted as part of a community-based intervention targeting nutrition and physical activity promotion among young and/or socio-economically deprived pregnant women in a regional population of ~500,000 (the Growing Years Project).

Case study: Strategy feasibility testing as a basis for intervention design for the Growing Years Project

Objective

To engage stakeholders in intervention design decision-making and to test a range of strategy options against a suite of assessment criteria; to support intervention portfolio design.

Method

Facilitated group discussions were conducted with two stakeholder/expert groups (nutritionists, n = 7; nurses, n = 11) using a process informed by the Nominal Group Method. This involved describing a range of strategy options based on earlier formative research. This description involved disclosure of the strategy's rationale and relevance to the Growing Years Project issues. Participants were invited to discuss the strategy options and their discussion was noted for thematic analysis. At the end of each discussion, participants rated each strategy option against six predefined criteria adapted from the National Public Health Partnership's portfolio planning process.

The criteria were:

Effectiveness – To what extent will the strategy achieve portfolio objectives?
Acceptability – To what extent will the strategy be acceptable to the local community?
Sustainability – To what extent is the strategy likely to continue being effective after initial resources are withdrawn?
Selectivity – To what extent does the strategy reach high-priority population sub-groups?
Timing (effects) – How expensive per unit of outcome is the strategy likely to be?
Synergistic – Is the strategy complementary to other strategies and agencies? Does it add value to other strategies?

These ratings and the associated discussion themes were used to support an assessment of the utility of intervention options proposed.

Results

Discussions in response to each strategy description yielded important information relating to existing interventions and work previously unknown to the project team. This has been important to considerations about project and service integration, helped clarify the range of key stakeholders in each strategy option and provided insights that have proved useful in intervention design. Results of the strategy ratings process suggest most support for the baby-friendly hospital initiative, pharmacy-based initiative, academic–practitioner partnership and group education strategies. Whilst the BFHI initiative rated highly across most measures, it was considered too broad and outside the specific remit of the Growing Years Project, other than as a strategy that could be supported. Physical activity guidance in general practice and fruit and vegetable strategy options rated lower than other strategy options and were not highly supported in group discussions. Discussions from both groups identified the importance of consistent education and advice relating to nutrition and physical activity in the growing years period across a range of services and media, suggesting the need for a more integrated and multi-strategy approach to health education and guidance at a local level.

Discussion

This process proved effective in helping predict the strengths and weaknesses of strategy options proposed and identified stakeholder support for local interventions based on practitioners' expert opinion. It also helped engage practitioners from outside the local community/ project. The results have assisted in the formulation of a strategy–intervention mix for the first phase interventions of the Growing Years Project.

Source: Adapted from Hughes et al.[74]

The ANGELO process

The ANGELO (analysis grid for environments linked to obesity) process is a method for prioritising settings and sectors for intervention. It is linked to the socio-ecological approach to health, with a focus on creating supportive environments for making healthy food and physical activity choices, supported by health education, social marketing and

Table 11.1   Prioritisation – changeability and importance

Changeability	Importance
Feasibility	Relevance
Sustainability	Effectiveness
Acceptability – by parents, children, professionals, decision-makers, etc.	Reach
Affordable	Effects on equity
Cost-effectiveness	Other positive effects
	Other negative effects

Source: Adapted from Stanley and Stein.[73]

skill development. The environmental approach has been shown to be successful at complementing health education in other public health fields such as smoking reduction and injury prevention. It can assist with reducing health inequalities by influencing population groups which are hard to reach by health education strategies such as those with lower educational attainment, lower income and language barriers. Environmental changes can also be more cost-effective and have more lasting effects on behaviour change because they become incorporated into structures, systems and policies and sociocultural norms. The ANGELO process is designed for obesogenic environments, the sum of influences that the surroundings, opportunities or conditions of life have on promoting obesity in individuals or populations.[70] This approach has broader applications to PHN issues than just obesity.

The ANGELO process can assist in identifying and prioritising potential behaviours, knowledge/skills/attitudes and environments as a focus for intervention design. By systematically considering these attributes of a problem, a comprehensive intervention with a mix of strategies for action can be developed. Prioritisation involves the analysis team reviewing the changeability and importance of potential behaviours and related knowledge/skills and environments.[72] The key elements of *changeability* and *importance* are outlined in Table 11.1.

Task 1 – Prioritising behaviours

After identifying potential target behaviours of relevance to the PHN problem through problem analysis, determinant analysis and intervention research, each behaviour is individually scored on importance and changeability. A scoring scale (1–5) is used and it is important to use the full range of the scale to make prioritisation of the behaviours easier. The total score is then calculated by multiplying the importance and changeability score for each behaviour. The totals are then used to rank the list of potential behaviours. All behaviours must be allocated a single rank such that if scores are equal between two behaviours one must be chosen over the other.[72]

Key target behaviours for obesity

Increase	Decrease
Active play	TV viewing
Active transport	Small screen activities
Active recreation	High fat/sugar/salt snacks
Fruit and vegetables	Fast foods
Whole grain cereal	High fat meals
Water	High sugar drinks (including fruit juice)
Breastfeeding	

Task 2 – Choosing related knowledge and skills

The next step is to list the knowledge and skills required for the identified behaviours to occur. When developing the list it may be useful to consider any myths and mis-understandings, as well as skill gaps. Once identified, score and rank the knowledge and skills using the same scoring and calculation methods employed for the behaviours.[72] Remember: when ranking ensure each skill and knowledge is given a different rank.

Key knowledge and skills for obesity, related to priority behaviours

Knowledge	Skills
Fruit juice – high sugar	Cooking
High energy snacks	Fundamental motor skills
Value of whole grains	Traffic safety
Value of drinking water	Using food labels
Appropriate serving size	Monitoring small screen activities
How much TV/small screen	Introducing and trying new foods
How much physical activity	

Task 3 – Choosing related environments

The ANGELO framework is used to choose and prioritise environments for action. The ANGELO grid divides the environment into size (micro and macro) and type (physical, economic, political, socio-cultural). The *micro-* (or local) environment refers to *settings* that individuals interact with (e.g. schools, workplaces, homes, neighbourhoods). The *macro*-environment refers to *sectors* which influence local settings such as education/ health/transport systems, the food industry, local/national governments and society's attitudes and beliefs. Within these settings and sectors are the types of environments:

- The *physical environment* – Relates to what is available: healthy foods in food outlets, opportunities for physical activity, availability of training, nutrition and exercise expertise, technological innovations and information.
- The *economic environment* – Refers to the costs related to food and physical activity: costs to the individual, as well as budget allocations for physical activity infrastructure and cost factors of food production, manufacturing, distribution and retailing.
- The *political environment* – Refers to the rules related to food and physical activity: laws, regulations, policies and institutional rules that affect individual and organisational behaviour.
- The *socio-cultural environment* – Refers to a community's or society's attitudes, beliefs and values related to food and physical activity: the ethos or culture of a school, workplace or neighbourhood or mass media/societal view of food and physical activity.[70]

The ANGELO framework (Table 11.2) is useful to identify the environmental elements for targeting related to the priority behaviours. The tool is used with analysis team members asking the four questions in relation to various settings. It is simplest to consider each setting in terms of barriers, but there may also be important facilitators or gaps (e.g. policy gaps).

After identifying the environmental elements that should be targeted in relation to the identified priority behaviours, score and rank these elements using the same process as that used for behaviours and knowledge and skills. Table 11.3 is a prioritisation table. A separate table is required for each task.

Table 11.2   The ANGELO framework

Environmental size	Micro-environment (settings)		Macro-environment (sectors)	
	Food	Physical Activity	Food	Physical Activity
Environmental type				
Physical – *What is available?*				
Economic – *What are the financial factors?*				
Policy – *What are the rules?*				
Socio-cultural – *What are the attitudes, beliefs, perceptions and values?*				

Table 11.3 ANGELO process prioritisation table

List of potential behaviours/skills to target	Score			Rank
	Importance	**Changeability**	**Total (I × C)**	
Increase breastfeeding rates				
Increase vegetable intake				

Key:	
Importance	**Changeability**
(How relevant is this factor and change?)	(How easy or hard is this factor to how big is the impact?)
1. Not important at all	1. Very hard to change
2. A little important	2. Hard to change
3. Somewhat important	3. Possible to change
4. Very important	4. Easy to change
5. Extremely important	5. Very easy to change

This process is designed to assist strategy prioritisation resulting in priority rankings through a process of consultation and consideration.

The ACE process

The ACE (assessing cost-effectiveness) process is a systematic method that has been applied to assess the cost-effectiveness of obesity interventions in children and adolescents in Australia. The process involved evaluation of intervention strategies in two phases:

1 Calculation of an incremental cost-effectiveness ratio from the incremental cost ($) per incremental disability adjusted life year (DALY) saved.
2 Applying judgement criteria to consider other aspects of the strategy, including the strength of evidence, equity, feasibility of intervention, acceptability to stakeholders, sustainability and potential for negative/positive side-effects.[71]

The ACE process applied a numerical classification system to assess the strength of the evidence. A more qualitative approach was applied to assess the other judgement criteria by listing the considerations under each criterion and arriving at a summary position.[71,75] A final, overall assessment was then determined for each intervention

Table 11.4   Decision-making criteria

Criteria	Considerations
Strength of evidence	Three levels: 1. Sufficient evidence of effectiveness (effect is unlikely to be due to chance or bias) 2. Limited evidence of effectiveness (effect is probably not owing to chance) 3. Inconclusive evidence of effectiveness (no position could be reached – only few and poor quality studies available)
Equity	Is the strategy selective? Does it reach high priority groups? Is the impact evenly distributed or does it have high impact on a few people or a low impact on many?
Acceptability	Is the intervention strategy politically acceptable? Is the intervention strategy socially acceptable? Who supports/opposes the intervention?
Feasibility	Is there adequate capacity to implement the strategy? Is the strategy feasible in the current context? Are there contextual factors that will interfere with strategy implementation?
Sustainability	What is the sustainability of the action? Is ongoing capacity and infrastructure required for the strategy to continue?
Side-effects	What are the positive side-effects of the action? What are the negative side-effects of the action? How do these side-effects weigh against each other?

Source: Adapted from NPHP,[68] DHS[71] and Haby et al.[75]

strategy to assist with prioritisation. Table 11.4 outlines the criteria used in the second phase.

Although calculating the cost-effectiveness of intervention strategies may not always be feasible in PHN practice, the consideration of cost as part of the judgement criteria is important. For smaller-scale interventions cost may be included as a component in the criteria. Key considerations include:

- How expensive will the intervention strategy be?
- Will it save resources overall?
- How are the economic costs and savings distributed? Do they come from the same finance pot?
- Is the strategy affordable?

Table 11.5 shows the results from the ACE obesity study for the intervention strategy 'A school-based focused nutrition education intervention to reduce the consumption of sweetened carbonated beverages', one of the 13 intervention strategies reviewed in the study.

Table 11.5 Intervention strategy appraisal example, a school-based focused nutrition education intervention – ACE obesity study

Strength of evidence	Equity	Acceptability	Feasibility	Sustainability	Side-effects
Limited evidence of effectiveness: • One UK RCT showed a statistically significant decrease in prevalence of overweight and obesity but not BMI • Two prospective studies showed significant association of BMI and fizzy drink consumption	Potential to increase inequality due to: • Lower SES schools having lower uptake • Location of schools in remote area • Higher non-attendance rate at lower SES schools • Appropriateness to non-English speaking or indigenous?	Issues that may arise: • Uptake by schools may be low due to competing programmes • Preference of schools for a more comprehensive approach, integrated into the curriculum and delivered by regular teachers • Poor acceptance by fizzy drinks manufacturers leading to lobbying the federal government against the intervention	Issues that may arise: • Will require high level of cooperation between state and federal government • Availability of adequate workforce • Competing programmes may affect uptake by schools	Issues likely to arise: • Ongoing funding required • Whether mean reduction in BMI and consumption of fizzy drinks is maintained beyond one year is unknown • Competing programmes may affect willingness of school to retain this intervention	*Positive:* Improvement in dentition due to • Reduction in dental caries • Reduction in household budget spent on fizzy drinks *Negative:* • Potential to increase stigmatisation and bullying of overweight children if poorly implemented • Increase and/or exacerbate eating disorders
Any implementation should be carefully evaluated	**Significant concerns**	**Significant concerns**	**Significant concerns**	**Issues need to be addressed**	**Significant wider positive benefits**

Policy considerations: he intervention is cost-effective in reducing unhealthy weight gain in children aged 7–11 years over a one-year period. Key decision points are: equity, acceptability, feasibility and sustainability. A significant effort would be required to ensure an adequate uptake of the programme by schools, particularly in lower SES areas.

Source: Adapted from Haby et al.[75]

Practice note

Setting priorities and making decisions need to be based on criteria selected and agreed to by the project team or project management committee. The draft criteria then need to be opened to the public and decision-makers for debate and scrutiny. Allowing debate and achieving consensus on the criteria illustrate the transparency of the selection process and help convince non-specialists and key stakeholders that the decisions are not biased or risky but are based on systematic analysis, bearing in mind the local context.

Key points

- To select and prioritise intervention strategies to address the determinants of the identified population nutrition problem appropriately, the risk or benefit associated with the determinant needs to be acknowledged. Whether the determinant becomes a focus of a PHN intervention should be a function of the measurable or estimated risk/benefit associated with that determinant.
- Risk refers to the probability that a hazard will result in an adverse health event while benefit refers to the probability tat a protective/promotive factor will result in a positive health event. Risks and benefits are revealed by considering the nature, likelihood and severity of adverse effects and positive factors on health.
- Strategy prioritisation is the decision-making task of ordering identified strategies to assist with the later development of a strategy portfolio. Strategy prioritisation is best developed through a collaborative decision-making process, where key stakeholders consider all the available information on the health problem and the known interventions to address the problem.
- Agreeing on priorities and selecting strategies for an intervention are complex tasks with several challenges and dilemmas. A number of tools are available to assist with systematic analysis and prioritisation of the strategy. Useful tools include: the Assessment Protocol for Excellence in Public Health, the Angelo Framework and the ACE process.

Part 3
Action

This section comprises four chapters representing the action steps in the PHN practice cycle. The action phase of PHN practice, represented by the bar connecting the intelligence and evaluation loops in the bi-cycle, focuses on planning and managing intervention implementation.

Chapter 12

Step 9: Writing action statements

Objectives

On completion of this chapter, you should be able to:

1. Describe the importance and relevance of developing well-structured action statements for PHN intervention management.
2. Explain and recognise the different structural attributes of goals and objectives.
3. Systematically construct action statements (goals and objectives) that guide action to address a population nutrition problem and its determinants.
4. Consistently apply SMART principles to ensure all characteristics of good action statements are incorporated.

Practical Public Health Nutrition, first edition. Roger Hughes and Barrie M. Margetts. Published 2011 by Blackwell Publishing Ltd. © 2011 Roger Hughes and Barrie M. Margetts.

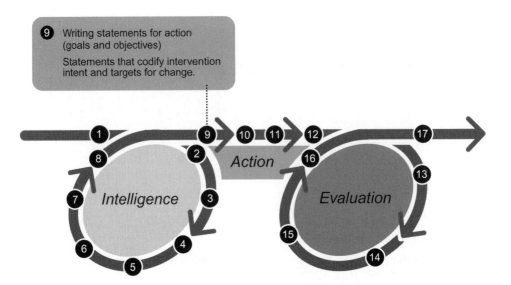

Introduction

Writing action statements is the first step in the second (action) stage of the PHN intervention management bi-cycle. The first stage of the bi-cycle (steps 1–8) involves gathering intelligence to define and prioritise the population nutrition problem and its determinants. The second stage is the process of solution generation, where the intelligence from the first stage is used to develop an organised and coherent mix of strategies to address or change the determinants that are causing the population nutrition problem.

Writing an action statement is the initial task in solution generation and guides intervention planning. Intervention planning is essentially the process of codifying a vision of the future (the intended effects of the intervention). Intervention plans are like blueprints and provide a logical deconstruction of the action needed so that the plan is transparent and clearly able to be implemented and evaluated. Planning is a collaborative process that guides intervention development so that it is appropriate to the identified population nutrition problem, addresses key determinants within the available resource limits and capacity to implement, and will have the greatest chance of achieving the desired change.

Intervention planning

Intervention planning is essentially the process of generating solutions. It codifies a vision of the future, the mission of the intervention, so that multiple stakeholders have a clear blueprint for implementation and evaluation. Planning is an iterative process, generating orderly, forward-looking action towards desired results. Intervention planning helps reduce uncertainty about the future and direct resources and effort in a coordinated manner to have the greatest impact.[76]

While there are no defined rules about how long programme planning should take, thorough intervention planning is essential to ensure intervention effectiveness and efficiency. Recommendations by Oshaug[77] highlight that intervention planning in community nutrition work should take a high priority in daily practices, i.e. planning should be prioritised over day-to-day activities.

Usual practice in intervention planning

Total time available − time for daily routine work = time available for planning

Ideal practice in intervention planning

Total time available − time for planning = time available for daily work

Note: Intervention planning in this context includes all the formative analytical aspects of planning (steps 1–8 in the bi-cycle model).
Source: From Oshaug.[77]

An *intervention plan* (see template in appendix 1) is a blueprint for the intervention and provides essential guidance for the development, implementation and evaluation of intervention strategies. Intervention planning should be based on what has been learned from analysis of the problem and its determinants, the capacity and commitment of key stakeholders and potential strategies for action. Careful collaborative planning and documentation of ideas and expectations of the intervention can enhance success and sustainability of nutrition interventions because the plan helps to focus and direct action.[78] The written plan outlines the key aims and methods of the intervention, a timescale of what is to be achieved, funding budget details, who is responsible for what task(s) and how the intervention will be evaluated and findings reported and disseminated.[76] Intervention plans need not be wordy or lengthy documents, but should be clear, concise and used as a tool for managing intervention activities. The value of an intervention plan is derived from its use, so it needs to be user-friendly rather than bureaucratic.

Action statements

Action statements are the goals and objectives of PHN interventions and state the outcome and impacts the intervention is intending to achieve. Setting goals and objectives is important for understanding the premise of the intervention design (the *logic model* covered in more detail in Chapter 13), and is essential to the development of the evaluation plan. Goals provide the framework for programme planning and must reflect the population of interest. Objectives provide a statement of the intended impact of the intervention and should be specific, realistic and measurable.[79]

The action statements for PHN interventions should reflect the nature of the change desired, be feasible and be based on projections from the intelligence gathered during the problem, determinant and capacity analyses. When writing an action statement, the desired level is commonly the ideal, and when what is technically feasible in the context is discussed and considered, more realistic statements are then generally agreed to.[5] Planning, therefore, often requires a compromise between lofty ideals and the realities of feasibility.

The development of goals and objectives should be based on what has been learned from the intelligence stage about the extent of, reasons for and factors causing nutrition-related problems within the community or population. Using this information, all the key stakeholders should work together to write and agree on the intervention action statements.[78]

Linking problem and determinant analysis to action statements

The determinant analysis created in step 4 (determinant analysis) has been used to define potential intervention points and understand what factors needs to be changed to reduce the identified population nutrition problem. The determinant analysis thus provides the foundation for writing action statements and clearly specifying the intervention goal and objectives. Figure 12.1 illustrates how the determinant analysis can be used to develop action statements – a useful tool for key stakeholders in the action statement development process.

The basic concept of Figure 12.1 implies that:

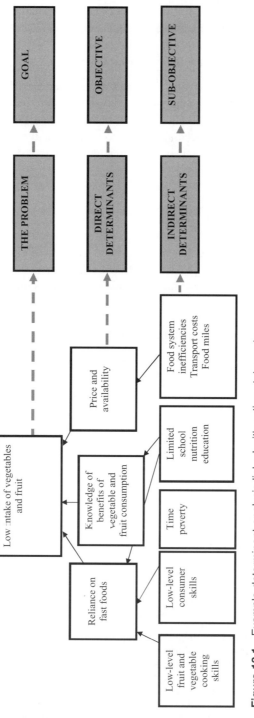

Figure 12.1 Example determinant analysis linked with action statements

- The intervention goal should reflect how to change the population nutrition problem – in this case increase fruit and vegetable intake.
- The objectives address the direct determinants.
- The sub-objectives address the indirect determinants.

Using the determinants analysis also illustrates an assumed causal sequence. That is, if strategies are effective at achieving sub-objectives (also referred to as strategy objectives), there will be a positive flow towards the objectives being achieved and ultimately the goals being achieved. Depending on the complexity of the problem there may be many objectives and sub-objectives, reflecting the numerous layers of determinants identified in the intelligence stage.

Writing intervention goals

A goal is a statement that describes in broad terms the desired direction or outcome the intervention will achieve. The goal should describe the general intent of the intervention and provide an indication of the value underpinning the intervention.[80] Many PHN interventions have a single goal. However, more complex interventions may have several goals.

There are a number of challenges for writing intervention goals in PHN, for example:

- Most data are disease-based (PHN is interested in promoting health).
- The field is still exploring intervention effectiveness.
- Accountability and direct measurement of intervention is becoming increasingly important.[79]

Whilst it is important to keep in mind that many funding agencies and decision-makers are seeking reductions in costly disease states (diabetes, etc.), PHN interventions should be striving to create positive, health-oriented goals. This ideological vision needs to be tempered by the political and organisational realities.

Intervention goals – key points

- A goal is the other side of the problem. A written goal is a positive statement of what would exist if the problem was no longer there – for example, a goal might be to 'reduce the number of premature deaths related to a high-fat diet'. Goals should be future-oriented, easily understood and broad.
- A goal is a statement of direction, general purpose or wide interest which reflects what changes in the problem are desirable. Goals describe what the programme will accomplish and is not a description of the service/project.
- As goals provide the programme planning framework, they need to reflect reality. The involvement of community and target group representatives in goal development is important. Goals can be categorised as short or long term. The development of meaningful programme goals is contingent on an accurate analysis of the health problem.
- Goals tend to be broad, all-encompassing ideals as they are derived from values. The formulation of general goals is essential because many of the most important human goals can adequately and meaningfully be stated only in abstract terms.

- Goals should be developed by the planning group by consensus (particularly among target group representatives). If consensus cannot be reached, then the planning group or goals may need to be restructured.
- Goals reflect the problem, i.e. if a problem is a lack of fruit in children's lunchboxes, then the goal might be to increase the number of children who bring at least one portion of fruit to school each day.

Ideally, goals should be written in terms of outcomes to be achieved, supported by measurable indicators. In some circumstances, innovation or a new approach is needed or there are conflicting goals between stakeholders, goals that state the direction of the intervention are agreed to. Goals should be developed by the project management group (project leadership or governance group) to reach a consensus (particularly among target group representatives). If consensus cannot be reached, then the group or goals may need to be restructured.

Writing intervention objectives

Objectives state the change that must occur for the goal to be achieved. Objectives are much more specific and precise than goals and should be stated in terms of actual results rather than in general terms.[6] Objectives reflect the determinants of the nutrition-related health problem. They highlight the most important determinants that need to be changed to remedy the health problem.[76] It is common for several objectives that reflect the determinants of the problem to be associated with one goal.

Objectives for PHN interventions must be tangible, recognisable and achievable within the available resources and capacity. Intelligence from the previous stage, particularly the capacity analysis, strategy research and prioritisation, should be used to inform the construction of objectives.

Objectives are concrete statements used to measure the effectiveness of intervention strategies, stating what is to be accomplished by a given point in time. Objectives provide the main energising and directive force for intervention action, and guide and direct intervention evaluation.[78]

Characteristics of good intervention objectives include specificity, credibility, measurability, continuity, compatibility and freedom from data constraints. The acronym SMART is an easy way to remember the key features of well-written intervention objectives.[79]

Ensure objectives are SMART

S – specific (describe the place, target group)
M – measurable (define an amount that can be measured in evaluation)
A – achievable (consider the circumstances and context)
R – realistic change (rather than ideal)
T – time-specific (time-frame provided for achievement of objectives)

Objectives are considerably easier to measure when applied to the SMART process. Once good intervention objectives have been constructed, the success of the related intervention action can be determined in a reliable and observable way by noting whether or not the objective has been achieved.[81]

Short-term vs. long-term objectives

Whether an objective is short- or long-term is relative to the length of time needed to achieve the programme goal. As a general rule, the time-frame for short-term objectives can be as short as 2–3 months or up to 2 years. The time-frame for the achievement of long-term objectives is usually 2–5 years.

Short-term objectives specify the short-term, or intermediate, results that need to occur to bring about sustainable long-term changes. For example, changes in knowledge need to take place to bring about long-term changes in health-related behaviours, or levels of support for a healthy public policy among decision-makers need to increase before the policy can be implemented.[79]

Examples

- At the end of the first year of the programme, 90% of teenaged mothers in Stockholm will know where to get assistance for breastfeeding problems.
- By the end of the first year, 80% of participating parents will have increased access to affordable, nutritious food through participation in the community kitchen programme and the bulk-buying club.

Long-term objectives specify the outcomes or changes needed to achieve programme goals, such as the reduction in the incidence of a health problem or changes in health status resulting from the implementation of a healthy public policy or environmental supports.[79]

Examples

- By the end of the third year, the incidence of breastfeeding cessation among teenaged mothers in Stockholm will decline by 50%.
- To reduce the incidence of social and developmental problems associated with poor child nutrition in Suburb X by 2002.

Process objectives describe what will be changed or implemented to achieve the outcome objectives.[3] Process objectives relate to the short-term or intermediate results that need to occur to bring about sustainable long-term changes. For example, levels of support for a healthy public policy among decision-makers needs to increase before the policy can be implemented.[79]

The development of intervention objectives should be a collaborative process and involve the project management committee, key stakeholders and, most importantly, the primary and secondary target groups towards which the objectives are directed. Objectives are more commonly directed towards secondary target groups to bring about the desired change to the primary target group specified in the intervention goal.

Example

- By December 2012, at least two of the following interventions will be implemented to enhance nutrition-related school health education:
  - Nutrition-related learning experiences are integrated into a course of instruction in each successive class level.
  - Training for teachers and other school staff on health promotion and nutrition education is health at least once per semester.
  - A series of extra-curricular workshops for students, staff and parents are conducted on preparing specific healthy and safe meals and completing dietary self-assessment.

Outcome objectives consider the changes needed to achieve the intervention goal.[78] Outcome objectives can refer to the educational, behavioural, policy, process or environmental outcomes the intervention will achieve:

- Educational objectives consider changes in knowledge, changes in attitudes and beliefs or acquisition of new competencies and skills.
- Behavioural objectives relate to changes in lifestyle behaviours.
- Policy objectives concern changes in existing or the development of new relevant policies.
- Process objectives consider levels of participation and working relationships or partnerships.
- Environmental objectives relate to changes to the environment to make it more health promoting.[76]

Example

- By June 2012, the knowledge of grade 10 students about the dietary guidelines will have increased 10% over baseline.

Types and level of change

There are several levels where change can occur in PHN interventions. Basic example objectives (not yet made SMART) are listed below and address individual-level, network-level, organisational-level and societal-level factors. These examples may provide a useful foundation for drafting objectives for PHN interventions.

Individual-level objectives[79]

- To increase awareness of risk factors.
- To increase awareness of personal susceptibility.
- To increase awareness of solutions.
- To increase awareness of health problems.
- To increase knowledge of ideas and/or practices.
- To increase recall about ideas and/or practices.
- To increase comprehension about ideas and/or practices.
- To increase knowledge of local services, organizations, etc.

- To change (increase positive, decrease negative, or maintain) attitudes.
- To increase motivation for making and sustaining change.
- To increase information-seeking behaviour.
- To increase perceived social support.
- To increase confidence about making behaviour changes (self-efficacy).
- To increase thinking about a topic.
- To improve skills.
- To change behaviour.

Network-level objectives (e.g. social groups, families, professional groups, church groups)[79]

- To increase knowledge of opinion leaders/champions.
- To increase prevalence of favourable attitudes held by opinion leaders/champions.
- To increase supportive activity (e.g. number of conversations about the health issue) by opinion leaders.
- To increase number and kinds of health-related interactions within networks.
- To increase favourable social influences/norms within networks.
- To increase social support for positive changes by network members.

Organisational-level objectives[79]

- To increase the number of gatekeepers, decision-makers and/or other influential people in the organisation.
- To consider policy changes or the adoption of specific programmes.
- To increase the number of gatekeepers, decision-makers, other influential people and/ or organisational members (or students, employees, etc.) who feel that the issue is important and change is necessary.
- To increase the quantity and quality of information regarding the issue and the policy change required.
- To increase organisational confidence and competence in making health-related policy changes.
- To change/implement policy and/or adopt/change.

Societal-level objectives

- To increase the importance communities and society attach to an issue by increasing media coverage.
- To increase societal/public values and norms (attitudes and opinions) which are supportive of the policy change you are recommending.
- To increase activity directed to producing policy change, such as collaboration among community groups.
- To increase the number of politicians who support the policy change you are recommending.
- To change/implement a policy.

Source: From THCU.[79]

Guidelines for writing objectives

The general guidelines for formulating an objective are to state it in terms of specific results, not in general terms. Objectives must be tangible and recognisable so they can be communicated to and understood by all those involved in planning, implementation and evaluation. Objectives must also be achievable within the available resources and context.
Objectives have four common elements:

1. the name or indicator of the nutrition problem being addressed;
2. the target audience (the primary or secondary target group);
3. a time-frame for completion;
4. the standard to be reached or the amount of change expected in either the indicator or the target audience.

There are two formulas to assist with writing good intervention objectives:

1. To [action verb] (desired result in the problem or indicator) [target audience] by [time-frame] (resources required), e.g.
   'To increase the proportion of parents of children at Stordalsbu Primary School who intentionally purchase fruit for school lunchboxes from 10% to 20% within six months'.
2. By [date] the following results [numerical[on [target[will have been accomplished, e.g.
   'By the end of Semester 1, 35% (up from 28% in 1995) of Stordalsbu Primary School children will consume fruit at morning break.'

Table 12.1 Examples of how to improve on draft objectives

Draft objective	What kind of objective is this?	How could the objective be improved?
To provide affordable, nutritious, accessible (easy to store, heat and serve) food to disabled and senior members of the Elders Village on a weekly basis by December 2011.	Process objective	This well-written objective might be improved by specifying the number of disabled and senior elders, thus showing the full scope of the activity. A related outcome objective would speak to changes in the behaviour of the elders.
Create more programmes that are geared towards promoting fruit and vegetable consumption.	This is fairly general and could be considered part of an overall vision, mission statement or goal.	To make it into objective it should specify a target date and audience.
To increase knowledge among young mothers of services available for breastfeeding support in X region upon completion of the project.	This is the core of an outcome objective.	This objective could be improved by: Setting a specific target: from x% to y%; and Setting a target date.
To increase the number of seniors accessing vitamin supplements by 300%, by August 2012.	Outcome objective	This outcome objective includes the four core aspects of a good outcome objective: target, population, indicator, date.

Source: Adapted from THCU.[79]

Key points

- Intervention planning is essentially the process of solution generation and creates a vision of the future (i.e. the mission of the intervention). Planning is a collaborative process and guides development of an intervention that is appropriate to the identified population nutrition problem within the available resource limits, and which will have the best chance of achieving the desired change.
- Action statements are the goals and objectives of PHN interventions that state what outcome and impacts the intervention is intending to achieve. The development of goals and objectives should be based on what has been learned from the intelligence stage, particularly the determinant analysis where identification of determinants and potential intervention points provides the foundation for writing action statements.
- Goals provide the framework for programme planning and must reflect the population of interest. The goal should describe in broad terms the desired direction or outcome the intervention will achieve and provide an indication of the value underpinning the intervention.
- Objectives provide a statement specifying the intended impact of the intervention and are stated in terms of specific results rather than general terms. Objectives state the change that must occur for the goal to be achieved and are much more specific and should be specific, realistic and measurable.

Chapter 13

Step 10: Logic modelling

Objectives

On completion of this chapter you should be able to:

1. Describe the relevance and role of logic models in PHN intervention management.
2. Explain the various types of logic models and the process for developing a logic model.
3. Apply logic modelling principles and processes in PHN intervention design and justification.
4. Demonstrate how logic models are used to focus evaluation efforts in PHN intervention management.

Practical Public Health Nutrition, first edition. Roger Hughes and Barrie M. Margetts. Published 2011 by Blackwell Publishing Ltd. © 2011 Roger Hughes and Barrie M. Margetts.

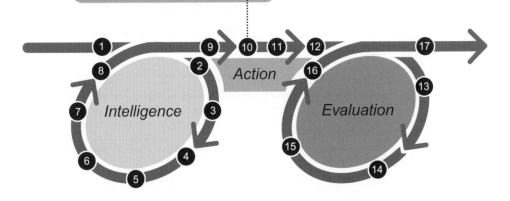

10 Logic modelling

The logic sequence that links an understanding of the problem, deteminants with strategies and evaluation measures. A conceptual device to enhanoe quality of intervention management. Includes testing feasibility amongst stakeholder groups to ensure strategies have support, meet needs and test assumptions.

Introduction

PHN practice has a strong focus on building capacity for effective intervention. Building this capacity often requires practitioners to have advanced grant-writing and other communication skills in order to communicate a vision for an intervention as a solution to a PHN problem. Logic models and the process of logic modelling in PHN intervention practice are very useful devices to achieve this objective. The age-old maxim 'a picture paints a thousand words' is particularly relevant to logic modelling, because the key objective involved in this process is to conceptualise your intervention in a diagram that clearly illustrates the strategy mix, assumptions and causal chain expected that will contribute to the achievement of goals and objectives.

Logic modelling is more than an exercise in drawing, it forces us to reconsider and make transparent our assumptions and the 'logic' underpinning our intervention strategy mix. This helps in the process of convincing fund allocators that the intervention as proposed is worth investing in and makes sense. This, after all, is what an intervention plan and submission are setting out to achieve.

What is a logic model?

A logic model is a diagrammatic representation of an intervention. A logic model shows the assumptions underlying the intervention activities and illustrates the association between the main intervention strategies, and the goals, objectives, target group, indicators and resources. A logic model represents the logic or conceptualisation on which an intervention is based.[82,83] A well-constructed logic model is like a road map or satnav route planner and should explain where you are going, how you will get there and when you have arrived.[84] The logic model will define the intervention outcome and boundaries, highlight important intervention features and show clear action pathways. Logic models are useful tools with which stakeholders can understand the overall structure and function of an intervention, and can be used to demonstrate accountability and results to funding agencies and stakeholders.[85]

Logic models are a core component of intervention planning. They are commonly constructed early in the intervention planning process to confirm the intervention vision and priorities, validate draft goals and objectives, and substantiate the strategy portfolio. Logic models contribute to intervention planning by:

- demonstrating how an intervention's strategies contribute to the achievement of the intended goals and objectives;
- identifying gaps and inconsistencies within an intervention;
- providing an effective communication tool;
- involving stakeholders in intervention planning;
- building a common understanding of the intervention assumptions, intensions and actions.[85]

Logic models are also a core component of intervention evaluation. They provide the intervention description that guides intervention evaluation by identifying what and when to measure objectives. Logic models direct intervention evaluation by:

- matching intervention strategies with associated objectives and indicators of success – providing a useful template for evaluation design;
- being a resource for evaluability assessment – the process of determining if a programme is ready to be evaluated;
- assisting identification of success indicators critical for intervention evaluation;
- showing funding agencies and stakeholders how specific programme activities contribute to the achievement of intervention goals and objectives;
- being a useful tool for engaging stakeholders in participatory evaluation.

Types of logic model

Logic models come in various shapes and forms, depending on the nature of the intervention and the needs and preferences of the stakeholders.[85] Although there is no standard format for logic models, they are usually depicted in chart form, with lines or arrows delineating the relationship between key intervention features (strategies, objectives, target population, partnerships, etc.), which are usually presented in boxes or ovals.

The display of boxes can be vertical, horizontal, circular or more complex and dynamic. The level of detail and use of cultural adaptations (like storyboards) are dependent on the complexity and context of the intervention.[84] Figure 13.1 shows a basic logic model layout linking strategies with objectives and goals.

Very complex interventions may have multiple models that interact. *Multi-level* logic models have linked levels displaying consistency of purpose and strategy across levels. Each logic model is built with reference to the level above or below it and is presented in a cascade. *Multi-component* logic models detail various intervention strategies and link the strategies within a comprehensive initiative.[84]

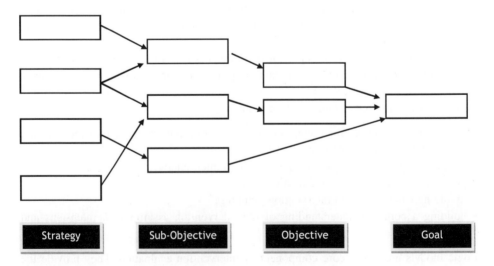

Figure 13.1   Example logic model layout

Practice note

Logic models are most effective when they are displayed on a single page. Constructing a logic model in this way ensures that only the key elements of the intervention are included and stakeholders can gain a more logical and simpler understanding of what the intervention has set out to achieve, how it will be implemented and what the key measures of success are.

Remember: a logic model should be a communication device and illustrate to stakeholders intervention characteristics of relevance, quality and impact and articulate why the intervention is important to them.

Logic model elements

In simple terms, logic models contain several key elements that are necessary to explain the link between the problem, the intervention and the desired outcomes. This may include a description of the situation, inputs and outputs and the outcome. Figures 13.2 and 13.3 illustrate the key elements of a logic model in two different models.

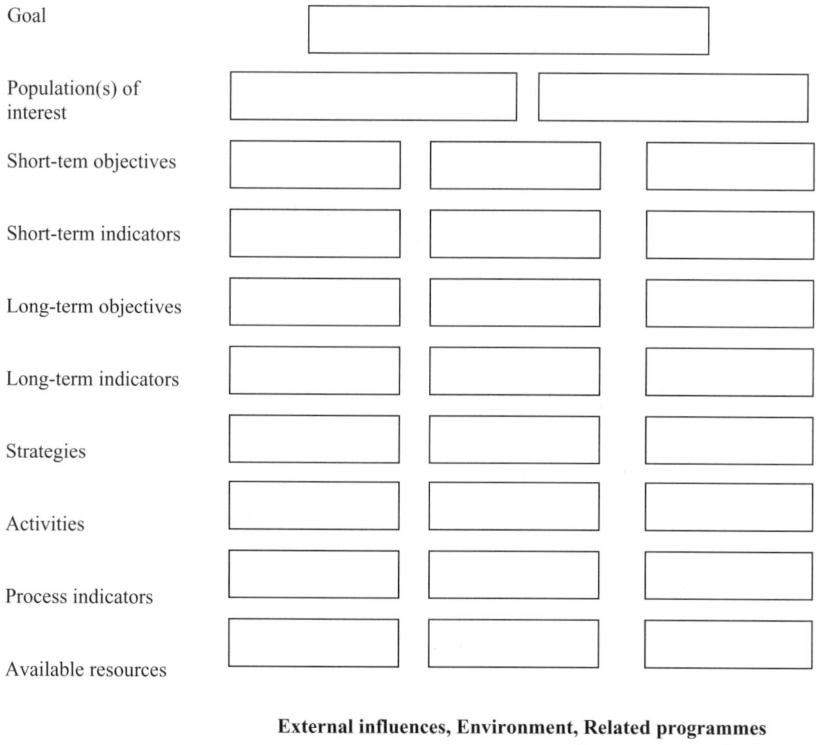

Figure 13.2 Elements of a logic model
Source: Adapted from THCU.[85]

Underlying a logic model is a series of *'if–then' relationships* which express the intervention's theory of change whereby the output from one effort becomes the input for the next one. A linear model may seem oversimplified as a simulation of a multi-dimensional process. However, the model can quickly become too complicated if an attempt is made to illustrate the reality.

Elements of a logic model

- *Situation* – The situation statement explains the relevance of the project, including a description of the problem and who is affected, and establishes a baseline for comparison at the close of the intervention. In some models this is stated as the *goal* and *target population* of the intervention.
- *Inputs* – The *resources* and *capacity* put into the intervention, including human resources (staff/volunteer time), knowledge, skills or expertise, fiscal resources, facilities and equipment required to support the programme and partnerships/collaborations involved in the intervention. Detailing inputs allows comparison of actual investments with planned investments which can be used to improve future programmes and justify budgets.
- *Outputs* – The *activities* and *strategies* of the intervention, including the populations reached as well as the action. Describing outputs allows a link between the problem and the impact of the intervention (intended outcomes) to be established.
- *Outcomes* – The results or intended impact of the intervention. Outcomes can be stated in terms of short-term, intermediate-term or long-term impacts and are useful to communicate the results of the investment. Intervention *objectives* and *sub-objectives* are often stated as the outcomes.
- *External influences* – Documenting the social, political, physical and institutional environments that can influence the outcomes. Highlighting the external influences helps communicate the broader supporting or hindering context and issues to all stakeholders involved in the intervention. External influences are not always included in logic models and may be replaced with process and impacts evaluation indicators.

Logic modelling in PHN practice

Logic modelling can be used in a number of ways to inform PHN practice, including:

- communicating the underlying logic and assumptions underpinning an intervention (as described above), but also
- engaging key stakeholders in intervention design and
- critically evaluating existing interventions (deconstructing interventions described in the literature into a logic model is often very enlightening).[86]

Logic modelling in PHN intervention management draws on the determinant analysis process completed in the Intelligence Module of the PHN intervention management bi-cycle, and provides the basis for the development of evaluation indicators (step 12: intervention and evaluation planning).

Figure 13.3 is a fictional example of a logic model in PHN intervention management and illustrates the link between determinant analysis and logic modelling.

Consistent with the community development and capacity building principles that should underpin effective PHN practice, logic model development should involve extensive consultation with stakeholders. Stakeholder participation tests the feasibility of the proposed intervention and creates increased agreement with the intervention design and participation in intervention implementation.

Developing a logic model

The recommended process for developing a logic model is to work through four key tasks:

- Preparing to develop a logic model.
- Gathering intelligence for the logic model.
- Creating a logic model.
- Reviewing the logic model.[85]

A brief outline of each task is outlined in Table 13.1.The first two tasks have largely been fulfilled in the first nine steps of the PHN intervention management bi-cycle.

Key questions for reviewing logic models

Reviewing logic models involves presenting and discussing the logic model with key stakeholders, then making revisions and taking action. The following questions can be asked in the process of reviewing to prompt discussion about the logic model.

Completeness

- Has the population of interest been identified?
- Are short-term and long-term objectives identified? Are they SMART?
- Are the strategies and activities linked to the appropriate objectives?
- Are there indicators for the objectives and strategies?
- Is there a mix of strategies across health promotion action areas?
- Is there wide range of resources and important partnerships outlined?
- Have all key stakeholder concerns been addressed?

Presentation

- Are there too many boxes?
- Is it easy to follow the arrows and flow of logic?
- Is there adequate blank space?
- Can the model be followed and understood by all stakeholders?

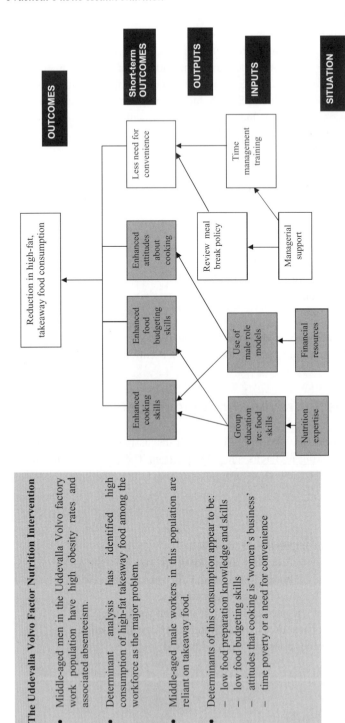

Figure 13.3 Logic model in PHN intervention management

Table 13.1   Tasks involved in developing a logic model

Task	Task element	Considerations	Relevant step in PHN intervention management
Preparation	Stakeholder engagement and participation Time-line Capacity analysis Decision-making	Logic models should be a product of 'collective brainstorming' by key stakeholders. Participatory processes can conflict with political and cost issues – set a time-line. Assess resources available. Clarify the decision-making process – how decisions will be made and who has decision-making power.	Community engagement and consultation Stakeholder consultation Capacity analysis
Intelligence	Gathering information and intelligence about the problem, its determinants and strategy options	Information to assist development of intervention goal, objectives, intervention strategies and evaluation indicators.	Community engagement and consultation Stakeholder consultation Problem analysis Determinant analysis
Creation	Decide how much information to include in the logic model and the type of model that will be used	The logic model must be meaningful, useful and relevant for key stakeholders. Determine the direction of information flow, the amount of text and visual layout. Try to avoid clutter and confusion. Review other examples of logic models.	Logic modelling
Review	Reviewing involves presenting and discussing the logic model with key stakeholders, making revisions and taking action	Review should involve assessment of: → Completeness → Presentation → Logic	Logic modelling

Source: Adapted from THCU.[85]

Logic

- Will the short-term objectives lead to the long-term objectives?
- Is the selection of intervention strategies logical and appropriate for the target group?
- Are the strategies likely to result in meeting the short-term objectives?
- Are there sufficient resources to drive the intervention strategies and activities?

Key points

- A logic model is a diagrammatic representation of an intervention. A logic model illustrates a sequence of cause-and-effect relationships between determinants of health problems, strategy interventions and outcomes to communicate the path towards a desired result.
- Logic models come in various shapes and forms, depending on the nature of the intervention the needs and preferences of the stakeholders. Although there is no standard format, logic models are usually depicted in chart form, with lines or arrows delineating the relationship between key intervention features (strategies, objectives, target population, partnerships, etc.), usually presented in boxes or ovals.
- Logic modelling is a core component of PHN intervention and evaluation planning. The process of developing a logic model applies the intelligence gathered during the PHN intervention management bi-cycle steps 1–9 to develop a graphical illustration of how the intervention strategies are expected to influence and address the determinants of the problem.
- Logic model development should involve extensive consultation with stakeholders.

Chapter 14

Step 11: Implementation and evaluation planning

Objectives

On completion of this chapter, you should be able to:

1. Describe the importance of implementation planning and evaluation planning in PHN intervention management.
2. Identify and apply a process for planning the implementation of strategies in a PHN intervention.
3. Deconstruct strategies into work packages that clearly define the work and resources required for implementation.
4. Describe and employ techniques for developing work schedules (time-lines) in PHN intervention management.
5. Describe and employ techniques for developing and designating budgets in public health nutrition intervention management.

Practical Public Health Nutrition, first edition. Roger Hughes and Barrie M. Margetts. Published 2011 by Blackwell Publishing Ltd. © 2011 Roger Hughes and Barrie M. Margetts.

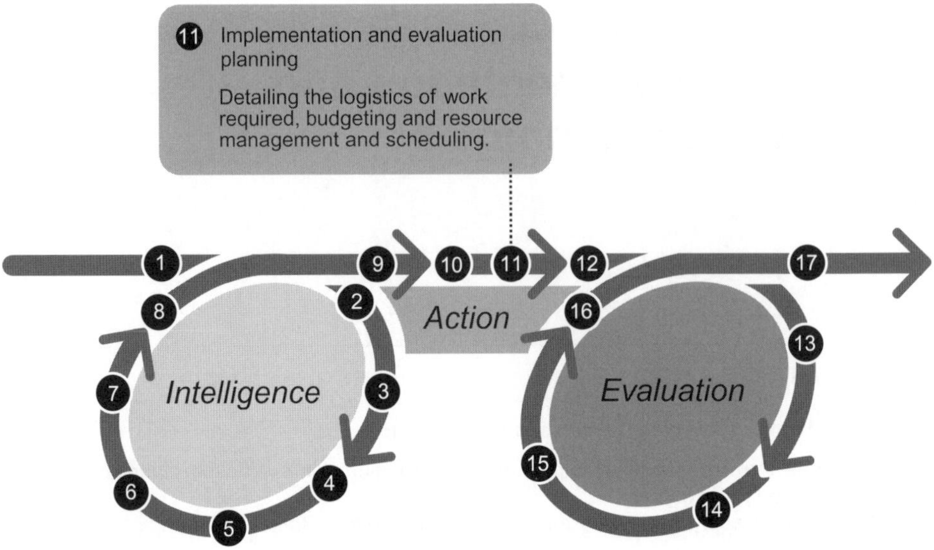
11 Implementation and evaluation planning
Detailing the logistics of work required, budgeting and resource management and scheduling.
1
2
3
4
5
6
7
8
9
10
11
12
13
14
15
16
17
Intelligence
Action
Evaluation

Introduction

Planning interventions (Chapters 10–12) focus on 'what to do' questions, but do not adequately detail the 'how, when, by whom and with what' questions important for strategy implementation. These questions are the focus of intervention planning covered in this chapter.

Intervention planning is a form of 'reverse engineering' in the sense that we start with a broad strategy structure and then break it down into its components so that we can identify which resources (time, money, expertise, etc.) are required to develop the strategy so that it actually works. In this process the implementation planning develops a blueprint for action. The blueprint should be sufficiently transparent and detailed to enable others to use it as a guide to strategy implementation.

Implementation planning starts with the strategy mix described in earlier action phase steps and systematically works through a process of:

1   deconstructing strategies into activities (or work packages);
2   considering the time and other resources required to do this work;
3   scheduling the sequence of work;
4   assigning responsibilities for work completion.

Detailed work packages are also key risk management tools because they force us to consider the logistics and detail of the work required to implement strategies, which often assists with recognising what may act as barriers and what we need to manage to facilitate effective implementation.

Evaluation planning should occur in parallel with implementation planning to ensure the two processes are linked – evaluation after all involves considerable work. This also encourages stakeholders to view evaluation as a crucial, inseparable component of the intervention that merits their participation. Evaluation assesses whether intervention objectives have been met, determines if the methods used were appropriate and well organised, and feeds these findings back into a planning process to improve PHN practice (adding to the intelligence base). The various levels of evaluation include formation, process, impact and outcome. Indicators are used as criteria against which to determine achievement of intervention objectives and strategies.

Engaging stakeholders in intervention and evaluation planning

In Chapter 3 it was argued that engaging stakeholders and shared decision-making were core practice approaches for effective PHN practice because it empowers communities, assists community participation in interventions and builds up the sustainability of intervention effects and actions. It is a capacity building approach. One of the functions of an intervention management group (a coalition of stakeholders to assist and share decision-making in the intervention management process) is to collaborate on implementation and evaluation planning. The key message here is to involve your intervention partners in the process described in this chapter. It shares the burden of decision-making, often identifies undiscovered capacity for implementation and helps keep partners working in the same direction.

The management structure of an intervention identifies the specific players, their responsibilities, accountabilities and the interaction between them for the life of the intervention. Ultimate responsibility and accountability for the intervention must be clearly defined and accepted at an appropriately high level within the partnering organisations.[87] Implementation plans can aid intervention management through the documentation of detailed intervention activities with time-oriented indicators. Intervention players can be kept accountable for their contribution and expected performance of the intervention activities, actual expenditure against predicted costs can be assessed and achievement of intervention milestones can be monitored. Documenting predicted activity for the intervention and subsequent monitoring of intervention activity enables project management to take if action milestones, budgets or outcomes of the intervention are not being met. Without an implementation plan good intervention management is impossible because detailed documentation for accountability is not available.

Planning for intervention implementation

Before implementing or putting the intervention into action, an implementation plan needs to be developed to identify and structure when, where and with what resources each intervention task is to be undertaken. Whilst the intervention plan describes how the population nutrition problem for a particular target group will be addressed ('what' type questions), the implementation plan details the specific tasks of the intervention identifying who is responsible for each task, the resources required and the time-line within which the task should be completed (the 'how, who, when and with what' type questions). Developing a detailed implementation plan documents the role of each intervention player and helps ensure the intervention is delivered on time, within budget and will be more likely to achieve the desired result.[76]

An implementation plan is a core project management tool (a blueprint for action) and provides a hierarchical breakdown of the work to be done for the intervention. Using the intervention logic model, an implementation plan considers each intervention output and illustrates in sequence, from general to specific, all the activities and tasks required to produce that output.[87] An implementation plan also defines the scope of work of the intervention – whatever is not in the implementation plan is outside the realm of activities for the intervention.

An implementation plan:

- Defines what needs to be done in the intervention and the order in which tasks should be completed.
- Determines resource allocation and define tasks for delegation and the skill set required.
- Confirms a common understanding of the scope of work among the funding agency, project management committee, senior management and the project team.

- Assists with identification of milestones.
- Assists with preparation of an intervention time-line (Gantt chart).
- Assists with budget estimation.
- Assists with identification of intervention risks by indicating areas of uncertainty.

Source: Adapted from TasGov.[87]

An implementation plan can be created using any techniques of listing and grouping project activities and tasks. Intervention logic models (Chapter 13) can be used to isolate strategies in order to reverse engineer. This essentially involves deconstructing strategies into activities and tasks (i.e. work packages) that need to be completed to enable strategy implementation.[87]

After a process of analysis (as outlined in Chapters 1–8), prioritisation and selection of strategies lead to the selection of a group-based food skills education strategy.
  The strategy is designed to help achieve the following objective:

- To enhance self-efficacy related to the preparation of healthy meals amongst single adult males.

(Self-efficacy is the belief in one's ability to successfully change behaviour and is proposed by social cognitive theory to be a major determinant of successful behaviour change.)

Table 14.1 provides an example of a process to identify activities and tasks related to each strategy. Generally, an intervention will require more than one page to complete this process. In brief:

- Write each strategy in a row, using as many rows and pages as necessary.
- Break each output into sequential units of work activities. Activities are all the things that need to be completed to produce the output and should be in the order they need to be started.
- Write each activity in a separate cell in the relevant output column.
- Break each activity into sequential smaller units of work (tasks). Write these in the same cell as the relevant activity.
- Review the list to confirm the activities and tasks are appropriately grouped and classified. If a task is adequately complex, it should be labelled as another activity.
- Check to ensure that completion of each set of tasks will result in achieving the activity and that completion of each group of activities will result in achievement of the output above. Move activities and tasks as necessary.
- Finally, give each item a unique identifier to use as a reference.

The table can then be used to inform other aspects of the intervention plan, such as determining resource allocation (intervention budget), developing a time-line (Gantt chart) and identifying key intervention milestones.

Table 14.1   Example of intervention outputs, activities and tasks – strategy 'reverse engineering' tool

Strategy	Activity	Tasks
Education group – food skills and knowledge	2.1 Identify nutrition expertise and develop session curriculum	2.1.1 Search local health networks for nutritionist 2.1.2 Approach nutritionist/s for assistance 2.1.3 Liaise time/resource commitment 2.1.4 Develop appropriate curriculum 2.1.5 Consultation on draft curriculum 2.1.6 Pilot curriculum 2.1.7 Refine curriculum 2.1.8 Design and print session material
	2.2 Identify resources and equipment for sessions	2.2.1 Identify budget available for sessions 2.2.2 Search and cost local venues/caterers 2.2.3 Seek quotes/availability from venues/caterers 2.2.4 Consult intervention team on results and confirm session dates and catering 2.2.5 Determine appropriate venue and caterer 2.2.6 Book venue and catering

Source: Adapted from TasGov.[87]

Developing work package plans

After identifying the activities and tasks required to achieve each output, work package plans for each output can be detailed. A work package plan should be developed for each strategy. In reality, many activities service the implementation needs of a number of strategies.

The details and development of a work package should be undertaken by the person responsible for implementing the activities and tasks. Developing work packages for intervention outputs allows transparency in intervention activities and identification of key milestones for each work package.

Detailed work packages descriptions are also key risk management tools, helping to reduce disruption if staff turnover or partner departure occurs as the details of the tasks to be undertaken are available and can be implemented by another individual or team if necessary.

Work packages can be illustrated in various forms and usually include specific reference to the sequence and duration of activities. One format for developing detailed work packages is the Gantt chart. Gantt charts are commonly used in project management which shows all the activities (and tasks if desired) of the work packages in sequence showing estimated time of completion on a horizontal car chart. Details about this useful tool are outlined in the following section.

Table 14.2 shows another format for developing a work package. The table lists the key milestones and major activities for a work package, who is responsible, the scheduled

Table 14.2 Work package schedule – example format

Work package ID	Task	Who	Scheduled start	Scheduled finish	Predecessor
WP 2					
2.1	Identify nutrition expertise + develop session curriculum	Project manager	5 February 2009	18 February 2009	
2.1.4 2.1.5 2.1.6	Develop, consult and pilot curriculum	Nutritionist	20 February 2009	30 March 2009	2.1
2.2	Identify and book venue and catering	Project officer	20 February 2009	5 March 2009	
2.2.8	Arrange necessary IT equipment etc.	Project officer	5 March 2009	11 April 2009	2.2
2.3	Advertising and recruiting for sessions	Project team	5 March 2009	23 April 2009	2.2
2.3.9	Final RSVP for sessions	Project team	5 March 2009	23 April 2009	
2.4	Educational sessions commenced	Nutritionist/ project team	30 April 2009	30 June 2009	2.1, 2.2, 2.3
2.5	Evaluation results reported to project management committee	Project management committee		30 July 2009	2.4

Source: Adapted from TasGov.[87]

start and finish dates, and the predecessor (if appropriate). In this format milestones are shown in bold and indicated by a blank scheduled start date. These milestone scheduled finish dates are determined when planning and developing the work package and are used to monitor the progress of the intervention. Activities in the predecessor column must be completed prior to the named activity commencing.

Work scheduling – developing a Gantt chart

A Gantt chart shows intervention activities and tasks in sequential order with horizontal bars representing the estimated time to complete them. The chart graphically depicts the time relationship of activities, tasks, milestones and resources in an intervention. It is a flexible document which should be regularly updated throughout the duration of the intervention.[5] A Gantt chart usually includes:

- the major activities and tasks of the project;
- the project milestones;
- the interdependencies between phases/activities/tasks;
- a time-line;
- the person responsible for each item;
- the resources required for each item.[87]

A completed Gantt chart can be used for day-to-day management, planning and reporting. It can also be useful to present to senior management and clarify planning estimates, work requirements and time-lines.

A Gantt chart:

- Develops a logical and timely sequence of steps.
- Assists in determining how long activities and tasks will take.
- Identifies the critical path – that is, the shortest possible path from the first activity to the last (useful for determining minimum time to complete the project).
- Uses as a baseline for reporting.
- Assists in determining how long the project will take, including analysing the effect on the overall time-frame of activities going overtime.
- Assists with identification of project risks by showing areas of uncertainty.
- Assists with the management of risk by showing the effect on the project time-line of a risk occurring.
- Confirms a common understanding of the project time-line among the funding agency, project management committee, senior management and project team.

Source: From TasGov.[87]

In brief, to complete a Gantt chart:

- *List the work/work packages of the intervention* – List all intervention outputs in a separate cell in the left-hand column, under each output insert a new row and list all the activities to be done to produce the output.
- *Identify resources* – In the resource name column list the resources required for delivery of the activity.
- *Identify who is responsible* – In the resource name column or in a new column list the person/team responsible for delivering the activity.
- *Estimate time-frames* – Use the remaining columns to create a time-line for the project. Estimate the time-frame required for each activity and fill in the cells in each activity row from estimated start date to estimated completion date. Order the activities sequen-

tially and in the output row fill in the cells from the first activity to the last to show the length of time for the output to be completed.

• *Identify milestones* – Milestones are significant events that act as progress markers for an intervention and are usually linked to the completion of a key project activity or task or may be linked to funding payments. Show milestones by adding a marker on the time-line (e.g. a black diamond or cell colour) and the finish date. Add a description of the milestone.

Table 14.3 shows a Gantt chart used in intervention management based on a simple spreadsheet.[87] The Gantt chart shows intervention outputs and activities listed against a time-line. Project tasks, the sub-activities that need to be completed to achieve each activity, can also be listed if required. This table can be used for a single work package or all project outputs. In some instances, the complete intervention time-line and the individual work packages (detailing the tasks) are all developed to provide a comprehensive implementation plan. The time-line of the Gantt chart can be in days, weeks or months according to the intervention.

Practice note

When estimating your time-line, be realistic and pragmatic about the expected/predicted time it will take to complete activities and tasks. Remember to take into account the level of input (e.g. a two-day task for a full-time worker would take four days to be completed working part-time at 50%). The more detail into which activities and tasks are broken down, the more likely it is you will have insight into the time and other resources required to implement the strategy. One of the painful side-effects of poor implementation planning is underestimating the resource requirements that leave you short of funds for activities you are committed to deliver.

Developing intervention budgets

Without a detailed estimate of the cost of each work package it is unlikely that you will obtain funding to do the intervention. Check the funding available and requirements of the agency/funder before you get too far down the road of developing the intervention; funders will only fund projects for a certain length of time; if your intervention takes longer to deliver, they will not fund it. By breaking down tasks and activities as outlined above, it will be easier to work out what it will cost to deliver each step/task and show the funder that you have thought through in detail the steps required to deliver the intervention. Budgeting information generally reflects funding for the life of the project; however, it can also be broken into intervention stages, work packages or financial years.[87]

Table 14.4 provides an example format for estimating the intervention expenditure. This costing of intervention implementation is a critical component of many of the economic evaluation methods outlined in a later unit in the intervention bi-cycle (economic evaluation).

A costing table can be developed for each strategy and then collapsed into a total intervention budget table.

Table 14.3   Gantt chart format

Strategy/ Activity	Accountable Officer/s	Duration	Jan	Feb	Mar	April	May	June	July	Aug	Sept	Oct	Nov	Dec

Table 14.4   Budget summary

Item	Description	In-kind cost *Existing sources*	Additional cost *Required from the project funds*	Total cost
Staff				
Catering/venue hire				
Travel				
Design/Publishing				
Phone/Postal				
Other costs				
	TOTAL	*Total in-kind contribution*	*Total being requested*	

Cost titles include:

- *Personnel/staff* – Wages, salaries, recruitment, benefits, payroll tax, on-costs and overheads.
- *Catering/venue hire* – Catering and venue hire for events, can include equipment rental, etc.
- *Travel* – All travel, accommodation and meal costs.
- *Design/publishing/printing* – Printing, publishing or copying brochures, invitations, reports, books, reprints, website designs and costs.
- *Phone/postal* – Teleconferencing, mobile phone, mailing costs.
- *Contingency* – An additional 5% of the total budget to cover things that occur unexpectedly. Be aware though that funders are wary of a miscellaneous column in the budget as this signals that the applicant has not thoroughly thought through the actual budget requirements and may have overlooked items of expenditure.
- *Income* – Including any income expected from intervention activities or funding milestones.

A costing table should include both direct and indirect costs. Direct costs cover the resources that are actually expended on the project activities. Indirect costs are in-kind expenses the partnering organisations are going to contribute to support the intervention. Indirect or in-kind expenses can include overheads, staff time, some phone costs, etc. Documenting in-kind costs is important for organisational finance purposes and because funding agencies generally can see the organisation they are funding is also contributing to the intervention. A brief description of the items and calculation methodology should be included (e.g. estimated hours' work required by hourly rate for different project workers). A budget summary table such as Table 13.3 is a useful way of submitting the intervention budget in a funding submission. Some funding agencies will set out the ways in which financial data are to be presented; it is vital that you use and follow the funder's guidance even if you may think it stupid or boring/irrelevant. Funders do not look favourably on applications that ignore their guidance.

It is not be possible to know precisely what each activity will cost, but the more research you do and the more detail the better; some funders require, for example, copies of quotations for equipment or resources, pay scales and levels of staff employed and time allocated for staff to each task.

- Get quotes.
- Have staff estimate the amount of time an activity will require.
- Ask finance staff to provide standard formulas for estimating on-costs and overheads.
- Use standard government and consultancy rates to calculate staff/consultancy costs.
- Compare cost notes with a colleague who has completed a similar intervention.

You need to allow time to collect these data – you should not expect that the finance officer will be able to provide you with what you need the day that the application for funding has to be submitted. In some settings you will need to obtain written agreement that the responsible financing officer supports the budget and that if funds are received, they will administer and be responsible and accountable for ensuring fiscal probity. If your line manager has allocated a budget for the intervention from within core or existing funds, they will still need to sign off the detail and ensure that best accounting practices are in place.

Practice note

Being able to predict accurately the resources needed to implement an intervention and justify this resource allocation is an important part of the grantsmanship process. A submission that fails to explain and justify how each item (e.g. salaries, travel costs, equipment) relates to the activities outlined in the plan is likely to be considered high risk and will generally not be funded. Remember to show 'in-kind' costs; funding agencies like to see the organisation they are funding are also contributing to the intervention. Accurate budgeting depends on a clear understanding of the work required to implement the intervention. Using the work packages developed that breakdown the intervention into activities and tasks serves as a sound basis for identifying and predicting the various interventions costs. Remember, it is important to be competitive when tendering for an intervention grant and consider how much your competitors are going to quote. However, do not follow competitors into making a loss – an intervention cannot be successful without sufficient resources.

Evaluation planning

Intervention evaluation is the systematic collection of data to enable critical appraisal of an intervention's activities and outcomes resulting in sensible conclusions and useful proposals to improve intervention efficiency, effectiveness or adequacy.[66,88] In simple terms, evaluation assesses whether the intervention objectives have been met, determines if the methods used were appropriate and well organised, and feeds these findings back into the planning process to improve the intervention. In addition to facilitating intervention improvement, evaluation produces knowledge that can enrich the quality of practice by contributing to the published and grey literature, thereby adding to the intelligence base. Sharing evaluation findings helps to inform future interventions, communicating to others the effectiveness of different strategies and enabling practitioners to make informed decisions when planning interventions. Evaluation can also help prevent the reinvention and repetition of errors.[76]

Evaluation starts at the planning stages of an intervention and continues throughout the life of the intervention. Implementation planning and the selection of evaluation methods to determine intervention effectiveness should occur simultaneously.[66] One of the flaws noted in health promotion practice has been the inability to build an evaluation plan into the intervention planning phase.[90] It is important to plan evaluation strategies in parallel with implementation planning to ensure that the two processes are linked and inform each other, and to assure stakeholders view evaluation as a crucial, inseparable component of the intervention that merits their participation, increasing the internal validity of the evaluation.[90]

Levels of evaluation

There are several levels of evaluation in health promotion and PHN interventions:

---

1. Formative evaluation – Data collected prior to the implementation of the intervention that are used to inform the intervention design and assess capacity for action. Learning from previous experience and pilot work before the maim intervention starts.

Formative evaluation is the systematic incorporation of feedback about the planned intervention activities. This type of evaluation helps to identify and rectify potential inadequacies of the intervention design and can be used to validate the problem, determinant and capacity analyses. Feedback about the intervention design may be obtained by conducting a pilot study or inviting critique from colleagues or experts in the field.

---

2. Process – Assesses whether the intervention (and various steps/tasks activities) was delivered as planned.

For each activity data/indicators/measures are required to show whether each task/work package was delivered as planned. It cannot be assumed, or implied without evidence, that the programme of work was delivered as expected. Process evaluation is critical to overall evaluation; if a programme is not delivered, it can never have an effect on the objectives (impact or outcomes).

> **3. Impact (summative, short-term)** – Measures whether the intervention objectives have been met.

Impact evaluation considers the changes that have occurred since the intervention began and how participants or target group think the intervention will affect their future behaviour. Impact evaluation commonly involves one of three methods: post-test only, pre-test/post-test or pre-test/post-test with control group. Pre-test/post-test design is useful to determine if a change in knowledge, attitude or behaviour has occurred, while the use of a control group helps to avoid the danger of overestimating the intervention effect by attributing all knowledge/attitude/behaviour change to the intervention. Results for impact evaluation are often expressed numerically from quantitative methods that increase credibility of the findings.

> **4. Outcome (summative, long-term)** – Measures whether the intervention goal has been achieved.

Outcome evaluation involves assessment of the longer-term effects of the intervention. It is usually more complex, more difficult and more costly than the other forms of evaluation. Outcome evaluation is important because it measures sustainability of changes over time and is commonly conducted (several years) after the intervention has officially ended. Similar to impact evaluation, outcome evaluation usually involves one of the three quantitative measurement methods to produce numerical, more credible results.[76]

> **5. Economic** – Measures the cost-effectiveness of the intervention or intervention strategies.

Economic evaluation involves identifying, measuring and valuing both the inputs (costs) and outcomes (benefits) of the intervention. There are four distinct types of economic evaluation: cost-minimisation, cost-effectiveness, cost-utility and cost-benefit.

Figure 14.1 illustrates the relationship between action statements and evaluation levels. Evaluation and planning therefore are interrelated and complementary.

It is important to note that evaluation is not an exact science. There is no absolutely right or wrong way to evaluate your programmes and there is no discrete formula that helps us in this process. People will have different opinions about what information is important. In more pragmatic programme interventions the measures used to evaluate impact and outcome may not be as precise as that used in efficacy research. Some consideration is still needed as to whether the methods used provide reliable, group-level estimates of outcome/impact, even if they may not be able to characterise individual intake.

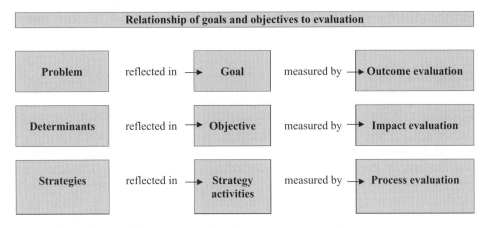

Figure 14.1 Relationship between action statements and evaluation

Key issues to consider in evaluation planning:

• What is the key purpose of evaluation?
• What resources are required and available?
• What will be the focus of the evaluation?
• What evaluation design will be used?
• Who will be involved in the evaluation process?
• Who will conduct the evaluation?
• Who will interpret the evaluation data?
• Who will have access to the result of the evaluation?

Source: Adapted from Ryan et al.[91]

Developing evaluation indicators and plans

Planning for evaluation involves considering two fundamental elements of evaluation:

1 Identifying a criterion or standard of good performance (indicator).
2 Gathering the relevant data through observation and measurement (focus groups, interviews, survey questionnaires or direct observation) to make an assessment.

Specifying the standard or criterion to be used to determine success is an essential component of evaluation which holds the evaluation process to public scrutiny.[12] Developing indicators is associated with intervention objectives and strategies. Indicators are specific measures that signify the point at which goals and objectives have been achieved and are used as the criteria in intervention evaluation.[13] There can be more than one indicator linked to an objective or strategy and often these indicators are measures of parts of goals and objectives that cannot be directly measured. The development of evaluation indicators involves using the intervention logic model to re-examine the objectives and strategies. Each objective and strategy should have at least one clearly defined indicator of success.

Impact indicators

Objectives may be divided into longer-term and shorter-term objectives and sub-objectives. Longer-term impact indicators are usually about attitude, knowledge, behaviour or policy change, while short-term impact indicators are the results measured as soon as the intervention is completed. The impact indicators that correspond with an objective should specify what information will be collected to determine whether the intervention has achieved its objectives. Longer-term impact indicators do not necessarily contain the degree of change required or the directions if there are no set standards, or previous findings to base predictions about the amount of change. Shorter-term impact indicators include reported barriers and facilitators to change, lessons learned from working with the target group and participant perceptions/knowledge of the intervention.[81]

Process indicators

Intervention strategies or activities could be reviewed or revised every three or six months, annually or biannually, depending on how long they take to be implemented. Process indicators consider the course of action and usually measure reach, distribution level, appropriateness of the strategies, ideas for improvement, participant satisfaction and feedback, etc.[79] The process of developing evaluation indicators and a plan should be consultative and involve participation from stakeholders and the target group.

Practice note

Evaluation planning should be heavily dependent on and integrated with determinant analysis and related logic modelling. Evaluation needs to answer the questions:

- Has the intervention changed determinants?
- By how much?
- How and why? (or, just as important, why not?)

Key points

- An implementation plan is a core project management tool and provides a hierarchical breakdown of the work to be done for the intervention. The intervention logic model is used to develop the implementation plan by identifying each intervention output and illustrating in sequence, from the general to the specific, all the activities and tasks required to produce that output.

- A Gantt chart shows intervention activities and tasks in sequential order with horizontal bars representing the estimated time to complete them. The chart graphically depicts the time relationship of activities, tasks, milestones and resources in an intervention.
- Budgeting is the determination of costs associated with the activities of the intervention. Developing an intervention budget involves calculating the cost of each activity. A costing table can be developed for each work package; in some cases a single, overall budget may be more appropriate.
- Implementation plans can aid intervention management through the documentation of detailed intervention activities with time-oriented indicators. Intervention players can be kept accountable for their contribution and expected performance of the intervention activities, actual expenditure against predicted costs can be assessed and achievement of intervention milestones can be monitored.
- Evaluation assesses whether intervention objectives have been met, determines if the methods used were appropriate and well organised, and feeds these findings back into the planning process to improve PHN practice. The various levels of evaluation include formative, process, impact and outcome. Indicators are used as criteria against which to determine achievement of intervention objectives and strategies.

Chapter 15

Step 12: Managing implementation

Objectives

On completion of this chapter, you should be able to:

1. Describe the various approaches to the implementation of PHN intervention.
2. Describe the importance and role of governance in PHN interventions and apply the key strategies of a good governance model.
3. Identify and apply tools for risk management in PHN interventions.
4. Identify and apply tools for monitoring the progress of PHN intervention implementation.

Practical Public Health Nutrition, first edition. Roger Hughes and Barrie M. Margetts. Published 2011 by Blackwell Publishing Ltd. © 2011 Roger Hughes and Barrie M. Margetts.

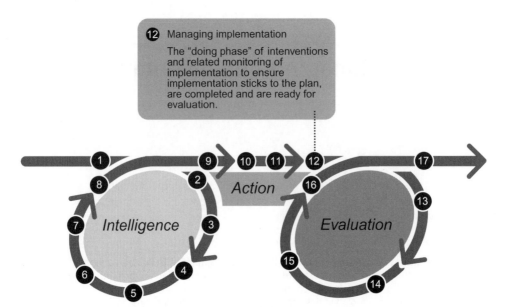

Introduction

The effectiveness of PHN practice is tightly linked to the quality and quantity (dose) of strategy implementation. Incomplete implementation ('implementation failure') is a principal cause of disappointing effects and outcomes observed in practice. Actively managing and monitoring implementation of intervention strategies to ensure that implementation occurs *as planned* is a critical stage in the PHN intervention bi-cycle. In addition to considering the implementation type, a number of factors, including governance, risk management, partnership satisfaction and evaluability assessment, should be monitored during the implementation phase of a PHN intervention.

Types of PHN intervention implementation

One of the risks in PHN practice is that so much attention can be devoted to analysing problems and developing objectives and strategies to address the problem that the type and purpose of implementation may be overlooked.[76] There are several approaches to implementation that can be taken, including:

- *Pilot approach* – This is an important first step in implementing a new PHN intervention and involves gaining feedback from a sub-group of intervention recipients and key stakeholders about the quality of all dimensions of the intervention. Piloting an intervention emphasises process evaluation and works to ensure the proposed strategy mix is feasibly and efficiently implemented. Intervention pilots are important to ensure that the risk of implementation failure is limited in later intervention rollouts.
- *Phased-in approach* – This occurs when interventions are implemented at different sites, communities or regions and rolled out progressively as circumstances (resources, time, opportunities, etc.) allow.
- *Immediate implementation* – Interventions that have been effective in the past or programmes that take a standard approach are usually implemented immediately and in full.[87]

A pilot approach is recommended for any new intervention because it serves to further engage the target group in the design, process evaluation and execution of the intervention, further securing commitment from the target group or community (i.e. capacity building, ensuring sustainability).

Practice note

Implementing an intervention can be challenging. Even with detailed implementation and evaluation plans unexpected issues or situations can arise which may throw implementation off course, requiring milestone or budget adjustment. Having a strong and clearly articulated governance structure that can be responsive to the changing practice landscape is vital to ensure decisions are delegated to, and made by, those with appropriate responsibility when issues or situations do arise. This is part of the benefit of having a intervention management group to share the burden of the crisis that will inevitably occur during an intervention's lifespan.

Governance

If we are serious about engaging stakeholders and building capacity for effective PHN action, it is vital that the management or governance structure of the intervention is identified and agreed to. The objective of intervention governance means shared decision-making to manage the project throughout its life, including the realisation of intervention deliverables, maximising productivity and quality outputs and appropriate risk management.[87] Management or steering committees play an important role by taking responsibility for the business associated with an intervention, ultimately ensuring delivery of intervention activities and appropriate risk management (i.e. issues are adequately addressed and kept under control).

Key components to effective governance

- Clearly defined roles and responsibilities – agreed to and signed off by the intervention management committee.
- A representative intervention management committee of appropriate stakeholders who steer rather than drive the intervention.
- Well-defined risks and issues for the intervention, including documented monitoring.
- Reporting of intervention progress against the milestones, as outlined in the implementation plan.

Source: From TasGov.[87]

Intervention management structures can be a source of conflict with regard to accountability and reporting, particularly when the governance structure does not reflect operational line management structures. It is therefore very important that all players know and agree with how the intervention governance structure will operate. Intervention activities should be managed through the intervention management structure, while operational activities should be managed through existing line management structures. The distinction between these two types of activities, intervention and normal business should be clearly conveyed to assist with defining accountability and reporting arrangements.[87]

The intervention management/steering committee

An intervention management committee or steering committee is often crucial for intervention success, particularly for larger interventions. Steering committee members play an important role in the intervention both individually and collectively. The primary function of a steering committee is to take responsibility for the business associated with an intervention, and ultimately ensure delivery of intervention activities and appropriate risk management (i.e. issues are adequately addressed and kept under control).

For management committees to work effectively the right people must be involved. Appointments should be based on skills and attributes rather than on members' formal roles, and members should maintain membership even if their role within an organisation changes. It is also important and desirable to have representatives from key stakeholder groups as members of a management committee (see Step 3, stakeholder analysis and engagement). It may be necessary to develop terms of reference to which the steering committee agree to ensure all members are aware of their roles and responsibilities.

In practice the intervention management committee's responsibilities involve five main functions:

1 *Approval of changes to the intervention and its supporting documentation* – Including intervention priorities and objectives, budget, deliverables, schedule amendments and risk management strategies.
2 *Monitoring and review of the intervention* – Including reviewing the status of the intervention at the end of each phase to determine whether the team should progress.
3 *Providing assistance to the intervention when required* – Including being active advocates of the intervention and helping facilitate broad support for it, facilitating communication with stakeholder groups, illustrating intervention benefits and contributing individual knowledge or experience.
4 *Resolving intervention conflicts* – Conflicts in resource allocation, output quality or level of stakeholder commitment. While the project manager should be able to deal with most conflicts, there may be occasions when the management committee are required to help resolve disputes.
5 *Formal acceptance of intervention deliverables* – The management committee should formally review and accept project outputs and are therefore required to have a broad understanding of the intervention and approach employed by the intervention team.[87]

A steering/management committee should meet regularly throughout the course of the intervention to monitor the progress of the intervention and address any issues that may arise. The project leader (often a PHN practitioner) should attend these meetings to act as a source of information and be kept informed about the committee's decisions.

Steering/ management committee agenda – example

- Introductory items:
  - Apologies.
  - Acceptance of minutes from last meeting.
  - Matters arising from the minutes addressed.
- Implementation plan business – amendments, revisions or issues arising.
- Intervention management issues – progress reports, consultant reports/findings.
- Important issues at the time of the meeting.
- Review of actions arising from last committee meeting – any follow-ups required.
- Plans for the next meeting.

Source: From TasGov.[87]

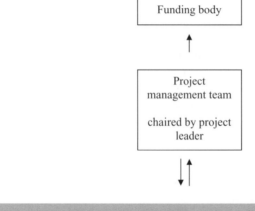

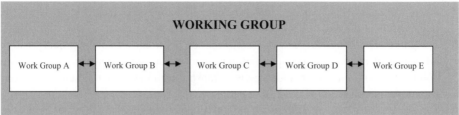

Figure 15.1   Example of an intervention governance model

The management committee has responsibility for the intervention until the deliverables and outcomes have been achieved, which may not occur until after the project team have completed their involvement.

Figure 15.1 shows an intervention governance model for a medium-scale intervention which may be useful to include in the intervention management committee terms of reference and implementation plan.

Practice note

In Australia, the governance model for the Growing Years Project (a Gold Coast-based, multi-partner, multi-strategy community intervention targeting nutrition and physical activity during pregnancy) included a project management team composed of core stakeholders (~10 individuals representing key partner organisations or jurisdictions). The project management team met fortnightly to monitor project implementation and share decision-making and information. Day-to-day implementation responsibility and decision-making were delegated to working groups, each with its own leader, and defined implementation budgets and plans. These project groups maintain regular communication with the project leader and other members via regular project management team meetings.

Managing risk

Many situations in practice involve decision-making in the presence of high risk, often due to imperfect information or personal preferences. A risk consists of two parts: an undesirable outcome; and the probability of its occurrence.[87]

Outcomes may be known or unknown. For example, the undesirable effects of excess fat and sugar intake can be obesity or diabetes, while the long-term health outcome of genetically modified foods is largely unknown.

Risk management involves progressing through five steps (see Table 15.1).

Table 15.1   The five steps of risk management

Step	Action	Description	Examples
1	Risk identification	Determining the possible risks of an intervention or faced by a population.	Project staff turnover.
2	Risk analysis	Determining the importance of the risk in terms of the probability of its occurrence and impact, as well as the expected effect of alternative actions.	Disruptions in intervention implementation, relationship building, salary budget, loss of tacit knowledge. Probability estimated through human resource staff statistics.
3	Action evaluation	Determining what can be done to reduce the probability of the event or to mitigate its impact.	Appropriate recruitment to appoint the right candidate, attractive salary package – professional development opportunities, performance management and career options.
4	Implementation	Ensuring responsibility for implementing the decided actions is assigned and the decisions executed.	Required actions allocated to the human resource department, project manager, project staff supervisor, etc.
5	Documentation	Ensure reporting of the analysis, actions undertaken and the outcomes to improve future decisions and for accountability to funding agency/senior management.	Documentation of planned and achieved actions in minutes, implementation plan or a risk register.

Source: Adapted from Kunreuther.[92]

Risk analysis can be undertaken by the project manager or project team; however, it should be reviewed and agreed to by the intervention management committee. People's risk profiles differ according to previous analysis and personal preferences.[93] Having risks identified and reviewed by a group helps to ensure a more objective, thorough process and a more effective outcome.

Practice note

Risk management can be reduced by undertaking sound problem, determinant and capacity analyses to ensure that the decisions made during intervention planning are more likely to lead to good outcomes. Identifying risks, taking preventive action and monitoring the risks in an intervention are important and should be included in the governance structure of an intervention. Identified risk should be regularly reviewed by the project manager and intervention management/steering committee.

Partnership satisfaction

Partnership development and maintenance are important aspects of PHN practice and important capacity building strategies to support interventions. They are an important mechanism for bringing together a diversity of skills and resources for more effective health outcomes. Partnerships can increase the resources available for an intervention, increase access to and participation of the target group, and create new networks with different sectors or industries.[94]

Most partnerships move along a continuum based on the degree of commitment, change required, risk involved, levels of interdependence, power, trust and a willingness to share ground. Figure 15.2 illustrates the partnership continuum and levels of partnership.

If partnerships are to be successful, they must have a clear purpose, add value to the work of the partners and be carefully planned and monitored. *The partnership analysis tool* is available for organisations entering into or working within a partnership to assess, monitor and maximise its effectiveness. This tool is extremely helpful for monitoring partnerships in PHN interventions and designed to provide a focus for discussion between organisations.[94]

Partnership analysis tool

The partnership tool is accessible at: www.vichealth.vic.gov.au.

The tool covers three activities:

1   *Assessing the purpose of the partnership* – Why is the partnership necessary for this intervention? What value does the partnership add to the intervention?

Continuum based on:		
• **Commitment**		*Networking* – involves exchange of information for mutual benefit and required little time, trust or sharing of ground between partners
• **Change required**		*Coordinating* – involves exchange of information for mutual benefit and altering activities for a common purpose. It requires more time and trust but foes not include sharing of ground.
• **Risk involved**		
• **Levels of interdependence**		*Cooperating* – involves exchanging information, altering activities and sharing resources for mutual benefit and a common purpose. It requires significant amount of time, high levels of trust and significant sharing of ground.
• **Power**		
• **Trust**		*Collaboration* – involves all of the above plus a willingness to increase the capacity of another organisation for mutual benefit and a common purpose. It requires the highest levels of trust, considerable amounts of time and extensive sharing of ground, as well as sharing risks and rewards. This type of partnership can produce the greatest benefits.
• **Willingness to share turf**		

Figure 15.2 Partnership continuum
Source: Adapted from McCleod.[94]

2 *Designing a map* – Visually represents the nature of the relationships between agencies in the partnership.
3 *Completing a checklist which defines the key features of a successful inter-organisational or inter-sectoral partnership* – Provides feedback on the current status of the partnership and suggests areas that need support and work.[94]

Where possible, the tool should be completed by partners as a group because the discussion involved in working through the activities will help to strengthen the partnership by clarifying ideas and different perspectives. Completing the activities can take several hours because of the variety of perspectives among partners and the time needed to reflect on the partnership and how it is working. The discussion that occurs around completing the activities will contribute to the partnership because ideas, expectations and tensions can be aired and clarified.[94]

The tool should be repeated during the partnership. Early on, the activities will provide information about how the partnership has been established and identify areas for further work. Using the tool again a year into the partnership will provide a basis for structured reflection on how the partnership is developing. For longer-term interventions and partnerships it is valuable to complete the activities every 12 months for continued monitoring of progress.[94] Ongoing monitoring and shared reflection on how a partnership is working is crucial to strengthening and sustaining relationships between organisations and achieving effective outcomes.

Evaluability assessment

Evaluability assessment is the process of assessing whether or not the intervention is ready for evaluation and establishing whether the critical preconditions for evaluation are present. Note that evaluability assessment is usually planned in the evaluation planning process, but is usually implemented at this stage. It is a key intervention monitoring process in practice. Evaluability assessment occurs in tandem with intervention implementation and provides an opportunity to assess whether evaluation is on target and enables a review of what is to be measured to indicate intervention impact and outcomes. Undertaking an evaluability assessment should avoid premature or inappropriate evaluation of a programme.

Preconditions for evaluation of PHN interventions[89]

- There is a rational fit between clearly defined intervention activities and intervention goals.
- The intervention is properly implemented.
- Partners agree on the evaluation questions that should be addressed.
- How the evaluation should be conducted and what should be measured are agreed.

If an intervention does not meet these preconditions it *should not be evaluated* until they can be met. Commencing evaluation without these preconditions will result in inaccurate and misleading results, which will defeat the purpose of the intervention evaluation.

Steps in evaluability assessment

- Identify the primary users of the evaluation information – what do they need to know?
- Define the programme.
- Specify objectives and expected effects.
- Ensure that causal assumptions in the programme are plausible.
- Reach agreement on measurable and testable programme objectives and activities.
- Reach agreement on what is sufficient evaluation.
- Make sure the programme is being implemented as intended.[89]

A worksheet (Table 15.2) can be used to assist your intervention team systematically consider evaluability assessment.

Table 15.2 Evaluability assessment worksheet

Programme goals	Identify primary users of the evaluation/ what they need to know	Articulate the programme	Specific goals and expected effects	Ensure causal assumptions are plausible	Reach agreement on measurable and testable programme activities and goals	Reach agreement on what in the evaluation is sufficient	Ensure the programme is implemented as intended

Source: Adapted from Hawe et al.[89]

Key points

- During PHN intervention management so much attention can be devoted to the development of objectives, strategies to address the problem and planning an intervention that the method of implementation may be overlooked. There are several approaches to implementation that can be taken, including a pilot approach, phased-in approach and immediate implementation.
- Monitoring the progress of implementation is important and includes regular intervention management/steering group meetings, risk management, partnership satisfaction analysis, intervention milestone monitor and evaluability assessment:
  - Steering committees play an important role in the intervention by taking responsibility for the business associated with an intervention, ultimately ensuring delivery of intervention activities and appropriate risk management (ensuring issues are adequately addressed and kept under control).
  - Many situations in health promotion can be seen as an example of decision-making in the presence of high risk often due to imperfect information or personal preferences. Risk analysis and management involves following a five-step analysis process to identify the outcome and probability of risks, taking and documenting preventative or recovery action.
  - If partnerships are to be successful, they must have a clear purpose, add value to the work of the partners and be carefully planned and monitored. The partnership analysis tool can be used to assess, monitor and maximise the ongoing effectiveness of partnerships.
  - The planned achievement dates of milestones can change over time, hence a milestone history monitor can be used to show how milestones have been rescheduled during the intervention.
- Evaluability assessment is the process of assessing whether or not the intervention is ready for evaluation, and establishing whether the critical preconditions for evaluation are present.

Part 4
Evaluation

This section comprises five chapters which describe the evaluation phase in the PHN practice cycle. This section focuses on the different levels and types of evaluation and the importance of sharing practice leanings via dissemination and scholarship.

Chapter 16

Step 13: Process evaluation

Objectives

On completion of this chapter, you should be able to:

1. Demonstrate an awareness of the importance of process evaluation in PHN intervention management.
2. Identify the intervention players and participants involved in process evaluation of PHN interventions.
3. Apply a process evaluation framework to PHN interventions to measure and improve intervention delivery.

Practical Public Health Nutrition, first edition. Roger Hughes and Barrie M. Margetts. Published 2011 by Blackwell Publishing Ltd. © 2011 Roger Hughes and Barrie M. Margetts.

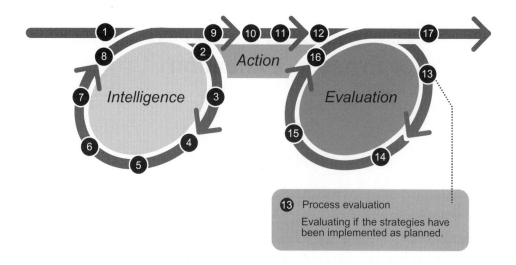

Introduction

Poorly planned and executed evaluation of PHN practice is a weakness in our discipline and a priority for workforce development. In practice, there are many pragmatic reasons for justifying limited evaluation effort (time restriction is most commonly cited by practitioners). Unfortunately, a failure to evaluate and disseminate evaluation results contributes to a limited sharing of intelligence and learning from intervention efforts. Evaluation and the dissemination of evaluation findings are professional and ethical responsibilities and we need to ensure they form a core part of our professional practice.

Evaluation focuses on developing evidence to support judgements about an intervention's success or failure. These judgements are often contextual and measured against levels and type of change defined in the intervention planning process (i.e. goals and objectives). Central to the logic of evaluation are accountability and quality assurance. Most interventions require access to societal resources (often tax revenue), so an account of intervention achievements relative to costs is a reasonable and often compulsory expectation in practice. Commitment to evaluation is a critical attribute of professional practice. It helps us build the intelligence about *which* interventions work, *in what context*, *why* and *how*, so that practice is improved and made more effective and efficient. Reflecting on professional practice and why interventions fail to achieve the anticipated changes required for health improvement is another important component of intervention evaluation. There are a number of levels of evaluation and multiple methods of collecting and interpreting evaluation data central to competent evaluation in PHN practice.

Evaluation – a brief overview

In PHN practice, evaluation determines the extent to which a programme has achieved its health outcomes and assesses the contribution of the different processes or strategies that were used to achieve these.[95] Evaluation of PHN interventions involves observing and collecting information about how an intervention operates, the effects it appears to be having and comparing these to a pre-set standard.[89]

The key reasons for evaluating PHN interventions is to assess and improve intervention:

- *Efficacy* – the effectiveness of an intervention under *ideal circumstances.*
- *Effectiveness* – has the intervention worked, i.e. has it achieved the desired effect *in real world contexts?*
- *Efficiency* – how well has the intervention done compared to other intervention options and relative to resources used?
- *Economic impact* – assessing cost-effectiveness and whether the time, money and resources were well spent and justified in terms of outcomes/effects.

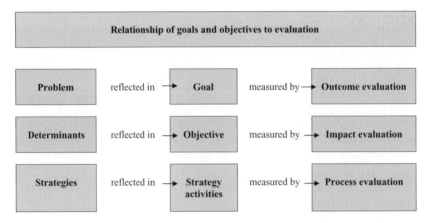

Figure 16.1   Relationship between action statements and evaluation

- *Intelligence* – the contribution to the body of intelligence to inform future planning and theory building.
- *Accountability* – justify intervention resource use and allocation to others.

Linking evaluation to planning

Intervention planning should be directly relevant to intervention evaluation (and vice versa) because evaluation needs to measure change in the problem and its determinants. The relationship between planning and evaluation in the PHN intervention management bi-cycle is represented in Figure 16.1.

Qualitative and quantitative approaches to evaluation

Both quantitative and qualitative methods are used to evaluate PHN interventions. *Quantitative methods* are derived from approaches developed in epidemiology, quantitative behavioural and social sciences, statistics and demography. Quantitative methods focus on numerical data that can be statistically analysed and test the extent to which an intervention brings about change in health status, health behaviour, knowledge, attitudes, etc.

Qualitative methods have developed from social sciences (e.g. anthropology and political science) and attempt to determine the meaning and experience of the intervention for the target group and other participants. Qualitative approaches include focus groups, structured interviews, participating with or observing target group members.[89,95]

No single approach is superior as the approach taken depends on what sort of information about the intervention is considered important and useful. Good quality evaluation usually has both qualitative and quantitative methods (i.e. mixed-method evaluation).

Practice note

Qualitative methods are often used in planning an intervention and defining the target group's needs, as well as identifying the barriers to participation and the strengths/weaknesses of the intervention strategies. Qualitative methods are used to assess programme effects and test the extent to which the intervention caused the changes in health status, health behaviour, skills, knowledge or attitudes. They are particularly suited to evaluating people's experience of the intervention and its effect on their lives.

Levels of evaluation

Several levels of evaluation in PHN interventions were introduced in Chapter 14. These include:

- *Formative evaluation* – data collected prior to implementation of the intervention and used to inform the intervention design.
- *Process* – assesses the intervention strategies and capacity building strategies.
- *Impact (summative, short-term)* – measures whether the intervention objectives have been met.
- *Outcome (summative long-term)* – measures whether the programme goal has been achieved.
- *Economic* – measures effectiveness of the intervention or intervention strategies relevant to costs.

Process evaluation

Process evaluation answers the question 'Was the intervention implemented as planned?' Process evaluation is completed before impact and outcome evaluation (which assess the intervention effects), as it is futile to expect successful intervention outcomes if the intervention has not reached the target group, involved the appropriate stakeholders or engaged with the community as intended. It is an integral part of evaluation to assess whether the different programme elements were delivered as intended.[89] Process evaluation assesses intervention implementation and is concerned with questions relating to intervention exposure, reach, participant satisfaction, delivery, fidelity and contextual aspects of the intervention. Process evaluation results provide specific information to help improve the implementation of interventions. Both qualitative and quantitative methods are used in process evaluation. Quantitative methods measure reach, delivery and exposure aspects of the intervention, while qualitative methods assess participant satisfaction, fidelity and context elements of intervention delivery.

Process evaluation is also of managerial importance as it provides rapid feedback on the quality and integrity of the implementation, identifying ways to improve delivery, resource adequateness and an understanding of the factors associated with success or failure.[95] Process evaluation techniques are also useful to monitor intervention delivery, even when there is confidence that the intervention is being delivered in its best form and is running as intended. Continued monitoring is a form of quality assurance by ensuring that the quality of the intervention meets standards of good practice and can also be used to ensure that the effectiveness of intervention strategies is maintained when diffused into multiple environments. An evidence-based PHN intervention, for example, may be trialled in one childcare facility and then implemented across a region to many childcare centres.[95]

Key purposes of process evaluation

- *Understanding and improving implementation of a PHN intervention* – Assessment of the quality and quantity of implementation activities, such as reach, fit with the target group and fidelity (intervention implemented as intended) can help to improve implementation of intervention strategies working to a loose plan and evolving in accordance with the context (particularly capacity building strategies).
- *Accounting for success/failure* – Identification of components of the intervention which have contributed significantly to the overall effects (distinct from the activities which were neutral or negative), and explain why/if effectiveness is confined to subgroups of the target population.
- *Enhancing best practice* – Findings contribute to improving professional practice by (a) supporting learning and improved performance within a population, (b) creating mutual understanding of barriers and facilitators among key stakeholders, and (c) building the PHN knowledge base.

Source: From Platt et al.[96]

Elements of process evaluation

Process evaluation can include a broad range of methods and measures; the most common elements are as follows.

Exposure

Exposure examines the extent to which the target group are engaged, aware of the health problem or receptive to and/or use the strategy, resource or message being implemented. Exposure includes both initial awareness or use and continued awareness or use.[97] Recall surveys are commonly used to assess the awareness of education or social marketing campaigns and materials. Members of the target population are commonly asked to recall the campaign and then asked to identify a specific advertisement after a range of different campaigns are read out. Monitoring exposure can enable intervention planners to take corrective action to ensure the target population and participants are receiving and/or using resources or messages.[97]

Describing or quantifying the awareness or the extent to which the intervention was received is crucial, as failure to achieve recognition and awareness of an intervention can have a profound impact on subsequent participants and intervention reach.[95]

Reach

Reach considers the proportion of the target group who are participating in the intervention and is often measured by attendance figures. To make sense of attendance figures the total number of the target group in the community, region or nation must be known. Reach data can be reported as a percentage or ratio. Percentages are useful for graphical representation; ratios (e.g. 1 in 25) are commonly used when describing an intervention.[89] Reach data can also involve assessment of the recruitment procedures used to approach and attract participants at individual or organisational levels and understanding the barriers to participation or reasons for dropping out. Undertaking semi-structured interviews or focus groups with participants and non-participants can help identify problems with access or attendance that may be addressed.[95] Monitoring the numbers and characteristics of participants ensures that enough of the target group are being reached, while monitoring and documenting recruitment procedures can help ensure a protocol is followed or altered as required.[6] Knowing the reach of the programme is important for understanding generalisability and explaining the subsequent effects. Identifying and quantifying any sub-groups who were less likely to attend shows low participation that will predictably lead to poorer results and indicates that additional services, different programmes or recruitment strategies may be needed.[95]

Satisfaction

Satisfaction examines whether participants (both primary and secondary target audiences) were satisfied with and liked the intervention. It is important to ensure that intervention participants enjoy and value the intervention before the desired effects of the intervention can be achieved.[89]

There are three main areas of participant satisfaction that can be examined:

1   *Interpersonal issues* – do the participants feel comfortable with the intervention? Do they feel heard and understood? Is it easy to interact with other participants? Are the facilitators interested, approachable and sincere?
2   *Service issues* – Is the intervention venue convenient and comfortable? Is it easy to access? Does the intervention strategy run at a convenient time? Are the facilities adequate? Is it too expensive to attend the intervention?
3   *Content issues* – Are the topics covered relevant and interesting? Is the information presented in the best way? Is the pace too slow/fast? It is too complex/easy? Is anything being left out or not covered in sufficient depth? *The importance at this stage is to ensure that the right topics are being covered at the correct level, not whether learning has taken place* (that is, *impact evaluation*).[89]

Measuring interpersonal, service and content issues can be achieved in a variety of ways, including individual questionnaires for participants, individual or group interviews and focus groups or group discussions. Individual questionnaires are often used, however caution should be taken to ensure that the group are literate and take well to paper and pen; adequate time is allocated; and all the questionnaires are returned.[89] It has

Table 16.1   Group discussion – community kitchens education session

Component of session	Positive comments	Negative comments	Recommendations
Content	Interesting Practical to daily life Good level of information	Didn't talk about reading food labels	Tell us where to buy cheap fruit and vegetables Include reading labels
Facilitating style	Friendly Not like a school teacher	Spoke too softly in the noisy kitchen	Speak up
Handouts/ recipes	Not too complicated Good recipes – the kids will like them	A lot of the information for kids not adults	A wider variety of recipes
Group work	Good to cook and eat together Lots of time to ask questions	Group too large for everyone to be involved	Need to limit group size to 10 members
Venue and facilities	Good location, close to public transport Good-sized kitchen Same equipment as home	Not enough chairs Too cold	Speak with management about heating
Other		Personal childcare arrangements difficult	Need to make childcare available

Source: Adapted from Hawe et al.[89]

been noted that positive response bias is common in this form of data collection, with participants giving unrealistically positive rather than accurate, constructive feedback about the intervention and facilitator(s).[1] Nevertheless, post-intervention questionnaires are often appealing due to resource and time constraints and are preferable to conducting no process evaluation at all.

Group discussions can elicit good process feedback, particularly with a less literate participant group. One such strategy involves the facilitator dividing a whiteboard or large sheet of paper into four columns (see Table 16.1). The left-hand column includes five or six aspects about the intervention (e.g. venue and facilities, intervention content, facilitators' skills, group activities). The other three columns are for positive comments, negative comments and recommendations. The recommendation column is important because people are more likely to give negative feedback if they can turn criticism into a constructive recommendation. The discussion can be facilitated as a whole group with the facilitator also making positive and negative comments, or dividing into smaller groups. Smaller groups maintain anonymity but it is important that the groups do not try to reach consensus – each participant will have her/his own thoughts about the strengths and weaknesses of the intervention.[89]

Obtaining regular feedback from the primary and secondary target groups is important to enable corrective action to be applied and the intervention strategies improved. Describing and/or rating participant satisfaction and outlining how the feedback was used to modify the strategies are also important to include in progress and final reports to explain to decision-makers and stakeholders why intervention strategies may have changed or progressed.

Delivery

Delivery involves assessing whether all the activities are being implemented as intended. Delivery usually involves writing down all the components of an intervention or intervention strategy and then recording and tallying the components' delivery and comparing to ensure all activities were delivered as intended.

Assessing intervention delivery may involve recording and monitoring the number of sessions delivered, the location and completeness of intervention delivery at different sites, or recording ways that intervention delivery differed at different sites. Delivery can also include assessing the running of an activity or event against a run-sheet for planning and implementation.[1]

The delivery of an education session should also be monitored for quality assurance and consistency. One method for monitoring content delivery is to have an observer attend each session and record the amount of time spent on each topic. After several sessions it is possible to see a picture of relative stability/instability and assess the emphasis given to each topic relative to the overall objective of the intervention strategy. Such monitoring can enable time adjustments, lead to improvements in intervention design and enable the dose of the intervention to be quantified.[97]

Context

Context considers aspects of the environment that may influence intervention implementation or outcomes. Context also includes describing the different settings and contexts in which interventions are delivered, and any contamination or exposure the control group had to the intervention.

Context can be monitored by keeping a log of problems in the delivery of the intervention (including variations in different settings), difficulties experienced or barriers to implementation. A sample of staff, stakeholders and participants can be interviewed about the environmental, social or financial factors that may have influenced the implementation of the intervention. For example, what happened when the resources were not available as required or the intervention was delivered to the target population in a way that was different from what was planned.[95]

Monitoring aspects of the physical, social and political environment and how they impact on intervention implementation enables corrective action to be taken as necessary and ensures the environmental aspects that affected the intervention are described or quantified against the intervention impacts or outcomes.[97]

Fidelity

Fidelity involves monitoring and adjusting intervention implementation as required to ensure theoretical integrity and quality of the intervention strategies and activities.[97] Monitoring fidelity commonly involves assessing the performance of intervention materials and components.

Methods for conducting process evaluation

There are various methods to undertake process evaluation. Saunders et al.[97] outline a six-step evaluation planning methodology which is heavily integrated with intervention planning (see Figure 16.2).

While there are no fixed rules about which elements of an intervention should be included in process evaluation, any clearly articulated components of the intervention logic model should be monitored[95] and all six elements of process evaluation should be considered for each intervention. Table 16.2 outlines the key methodological components to consider in process evaluation.

The initial responsibility in process evaluation when developing an intervention is to devise systems to assess the six elements: the exposure, reach, satisfaction, delivery, fidelity and context of the intervention and its key components. The information should then be used to make changes to the intervention strategies, evaluating these changes in a continuation of process evaluation until the intervention has reached an optimum and stable form. This is the time to proceed to impact and outcome evaluation.[89] Some monitoring of the process of intervention delivery is still required to ensure that the quality of the intervention does not falter. Some low-level continuous and occasional monitoring will help to keep the quality in check. It is important, for example, to continue to collect figures on attendance or intervention reach to track whether intervention reach has been maintained or improved. The aspects of process evaluation that are harder to collect (e.g. monitoring session content or intervention materials and components) should be monitored on a more occasional basis but not less than once a year.[89]

If an imported intervention is being implemented it is important to think of it as a new intervention because it is being delivered to a new group of people, by new staff. An imported intervention requires comprehensive process evaluation followed by scaled-down monitoring once the intervention is being delivered satisfactorily.[89]

Process evaluation indicators

Evaluation involves measurement and comparison of the observations or data against a criterion or standard. In PHN it can be difficult to be prescriptive because experience is

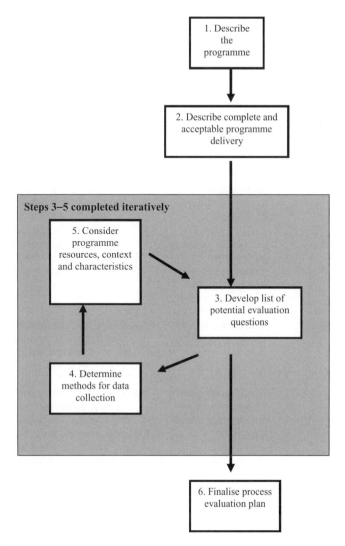

Figure 16.2 Six steps in process evaluation
Source: Adapted from Saunders et al.[97]

limited and emerging and because, commonly, decision-makers are reluctant to have black-and-white performance indicators for which they are accountable when evidence of intervention effectiveness is weak.

It has been suggested that it is appropriate for evaluation indicators to come from:

• historical comparisons with similar efforts in the past;
• comparisons with contemporary activities elsewhere;
• consensus among professionals which apply a combination of the first two and professional judgement.[89]

Table 16.2 Key methodological components in the evaluation process

Methodological component	General definition	Example – qualitative and quantitative methods
Design	Timing of data collection: when and how often data will be collected	Observe classroom activities at least twice per semester with at least two weeks' observation Conduct focus groups in the last month of the intervention
Data sources	Source of information (who will be surveyed, observed, interviewed)	Qualitative and quantitative – data sources include participants, teachers/staff delivering sessions records, the environment, etc.
Data collection tools/ measures	Instruments, tools and guides used for gathering process evaluation data	Qualitative and quantitative – tools include surveys, checklists, observations forms, interview guides, etc.
Data collection procedures	Protocols for how the data collection tool will be administered	Detailed description of how to do quantitative/qualitative classroom observation, face-to-face or phone interview, mailed survey, focus group, etc.
Data management	Procedures for getting data from field and entered plus quality checks	Staff hand in participant sheets weekly, evaluation coordinator collects and checks surveys and gives them to data entry staff Interviews transcribed and tapes submitted at the end of the month
Data analysis	Statistical and/or qualitative methods to analyse or summarise data	Statistical analysis and software that will be used to analyse the quantitative data Types of qualitative analysis used

Source: From Hawe et al.[89]

Data from process evaluations are often not published, so it may be hard to find comparative data. When comparative data are lacking, professional judgement and expert opinion should be applied.

Practice note

It is important professionally and ethically to obtain informed consent from all participants. Sometimes (e.g. observations at public events) obtaining direct consent may be impossible, however, it is important to ensure all participants are aware that data will be gathered by both formal and informal methods and not only surveys and taped interviews. It is also critical to ensure anonymity of respondents and confidentiality of the data and ensure that any reporting of contentious issues of a personal nature are handled with extreme sensitivity.

Table 16.3 Examples of process evaluation used in published health promotion papers

Author/(year)	Programme description	Types of process evaluation	Main findings and usefulness of process evaluation to this health promotion intervention
Ronda et al. (2004)	Dutch regional heart disease prevention project, Maastricht region	Steering committee interviewed: number of planning meetings held, count number of project activities held	Defined limitations to functioning of neighbourhood committees (understaffed); stakeholders rated community participation as 'not very good' and environmental strategies as 'not implemented'; these interviews helped make sense of the lack of outcome effects of the programme; may take longer (years) to engage with communities.
Steenhuis et al. (2004)	Evaluation of environmental change to nutrition strategies at worksites and marketing of healthy food choices at supermarkets	Interviews with supermarket managers about the healthy nutrition marketing and labelling programme	Most managers had a 'positive opinion', but indicated that health choice posters were the wrong size, labelling was not compatible with supermarket systems, programme materials were not always displayed, there was insufficient staff time and space in supermarkets, and the programme did not attract customers' attention enough –hence the programme's ineffectiveness.
Baranowski & Stables (2000)	Process evaluation of five-a-day fruit and vegetable project in nine sites in the USA	Monitored each project with respect to recruiting participants, keeping participants, context of interventions, resources used, degree of programme implementation, programme reach and barriers	Settings identified – schools, worksites; participation rates often lower than expected; in-school curricula were well implemented; worksite programmes reached blue-collar workers less well; programmes using social support, social networks or church-based networks showed good population reach; more research needed to define the quality of the implementation.

Source: Adapted from Nutbeam and Bauman.[95]

Process evaluation in practice – some published examples

Table 16.3 outlines three published PHN interventions where process evaluation has been an important and identified feature. The diversity of styles and purposes of process evaluation are well illustrated in these examples.

Key points

- Both quantitative and qualitative methods are used to evaluate PHN interventions. Quantitative methods test the extent to which an intervention causes change in health status, health behaviour, knowledge, attitude, etc. While qualitative methods attempt to determine the meaning and experience of the intervention for the target group and other participants.
- Process evaluation assesses intervention implementation including exposure, reach, participation satisfaction, delivery, fidelity and context aspects of the intervention. Process evaluation results provide specific information to help improve the intervention into a more effective form.
- Process evaluation is a continual process with intensive process evaluation to make changes to the intervention strategies, and then evaluating these changes until the intervention has reached an optimum and stable form before proceeding to impact and outcome evaluation. Some low-level continuous monitoring of the intervention delivery is still required for quality assurance.
- Process evaluation occurs before impact and outcome evaluation (which assesses intervention effects) because it is essential to identify, if an intervention has been successful or unsuccessful, *how* it worked, provide explanatory information and understand the mechanisms of operation.

Chapter 17

Step 14: Impact and outcome evaluation

Objectives

On completion of this chapter, you should be able to:

1. Describe the importance of impact and outcome evaluation in PHN intervention management.
2. Explain the difference between impact and outcome evaluation.
3. Apply an impact evaluation framework to PHN interventions to measure achievement of intervention objectives.
4. Apply an outcome evaluation framework to PHN interventions to measure achievement of intervention goals.

Practical Public Health Nutrition, first edition. Roger Hughes and Barrie M. Margetts. Published 2011 by Blackwell Publishing Ltd. © 2011 Roger Hughes and Barrie M. Margetts.

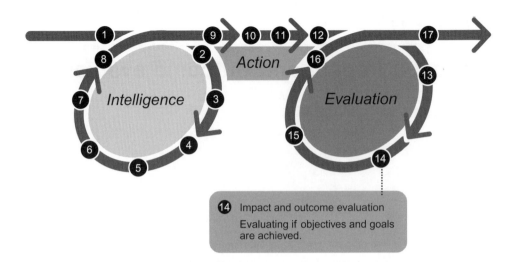

Introduction

Impact and outcome evaluation involve measuring the effects of an intervention and investigating the direction and degree of change. Impact and outcome evaluation test the proposed intervention logic model by examining change in the identified determinants of the nutrition problem, such as behaviour, attitudes, health status and environmental and societal factors. Impact evaluation is concerned with the assessment of the immediate effects of the intervention and usually corresponds to the measurement of intervention objectives. Outcome evaluation is concerned with measuring the longer-term effects of the intervention and this usually corresponds to the intervention goal. The key difference between impact and outcome evaluation is not what is being measured but rather is defined by the sequence of measurement. Whether a factor is measured in impact or outcome evaluation is entirely dependent on the casual chain of events postulated and what aspects of this chain the intervention is aiming to address. In this chapter the process of completing impact and outcome evaluations is outlined. Various tools to assist with measuring evaluation indicators, design types and technical considerations required for evaluation are explained.

Impact and outcome evaluation – what is the difference?

Impact and outcome evaluation both involve the assessment of intervention effects but at different levels. Impact evaluation is concerned with the assessment of the immediate effects of the intervention and usually corresponds to the measurement of the intervention objective. Outcome evaluation is concerned with measuring the longer-term effects of the intervention and this usually corresponds to the intervention goal.[89] For example, a community-based nutrition intervention may be attempting to increase knowledge, awareness and availability of fruit and vegetables with the goal of increasing fruit and vegetable intake by an average of one serving a day across the community. Impact evaluation would assess changes in knowledge, awareness and availability of fruit and vegetables while outcome evaluation would measure variation in fruit and vegetable intake.

Impact and outcome evaluations test the causal chain of events (logic model) that has been postulated by the intervention (e.g. that changing knowledge, awareness and availability will lead to a change in dietary behaviour). The key difference between impact and outcome evaluation is not what is being measured but what is defined by the sequence of measurement. Whether a factor is measured in impact or outcome evaluation is entirely dependent on the causal chain of events postulated and what aspects of this causal chain the intervention is aiming to address.[98]

A factor assessed in outcome evaluation in one intervention may be assessed as part of impact evaluation in another. For example, a public health nutritionist working in community health may be trying to affect change in knowledge and availability of fruit and vegetables (impact) with the goal of increasing average intake by one serving (outcome), while at the national or pan-European level increasing fruit and vegetable intake (impact) may be an objective towards achieving the goal of reducing the prevalence of obesity. It is important not to generalise thinking that intervention goals and

outcome indicators have to be stated in terms of health status, as is sometimes suggested.[89] PHN interventions at all levels should follow through the factors in the causal
chain they are trying to address by measuring both the immediate effects (impact) and
the subsequent effects (outcome) no matter what factors are being measured at each point.
If interventions were restricted to the assessment of immediate effects only, intervention
success would become narrowly and prematurely defined. Thorough impact and outcome
evaluation are needed to determine when the causal theory does and does not hold.[89]

With some interventions or intervention strategies, impact and outcome evaluation will
be focused on what the project management committee or community consider success
to be and how it will be brought about. This type of success measure is particularly
appropriate in capacity building interventions and strategies and may include changes in
perceived power and community self-confidence, concern for local issues or the formation of action groups. These are often important causal events and are the prerequisites
to other change. (Methods for measuring community capacity gains are addressed in
more detail in Chapter 18.)

When to evaluate?

Predicting when the intervention effect(s) will take place and the timing of the impact
and outcome evaluation are very important because measuring effects too early or too
late will deliver inaccurate findings about the intervention's effectiveness.[89] Hawe et al.[89]
suggest several possible effects an intervention can have over time:

- *Ideal effect* – the intervention has an immediate improvement in the nutrition factor of
  interest which is sustained over time.
- *Sleeper effect* – the intervention impact is not detected until some time after implementation such that the effect would be missed if evaluation is undertaken immediately
  or after only a short while.
- *Backsliding effect* – the effect of the intervention is immediate but only short-term.
  The effect would be missed if measured some time after implementation.
- *Trigger effect* – an intervention which triggers or brings forward a behaviour or event
  that would have happened anyway. Effects are seen immediately after implementation,
  then drop below the baseline level before returning to the normal or baseline level.
- *Historical effect* – cases where a health behaviour or target factor is gradually improving across time such that the evaluation captures this effect and wrongly attributes it
  to the intervention. This highlights the need for external or secular trends to be distin-
  guished from intervention effects (often by including data from a control community
  for comparison).
- *Backlash effect* – occurs when premature cessation of an intervention demoralises or
  disillusions participants leading to levels of behaviours or problems that are worse than
  baseline. Immediate evaluation would miss the subsequent negative effects.[89]

In order to be informed about which sort of effect may apply to your intervention
it is important to consult the literature for previous or similar interventions with a
similar target population and seriously consider the potential and likely effect the

intervention will have. Is the intervention likely to have an immediate effect that could taper off or is it likely to take time to show the intended effect? If predicting the likely effect is guesswork, a pilot study should be implemented with multiple measures over time to elicit a predicted effect and assist with implementing the main intervention.[89]

Key measures of impact and outcome evaluation

There are some common measures used in impact and outcome evaluation in PHN interventions. A mix of qualitative and quantitative methods is used in these evaluation measures. Qualitative methods interpret the meaning of the intervention for participants, staff, key stakeholders and those not reached by the intervention,[89] and are largely unstructured and observational. Quantitative methods systematically measures the size of the intended effects of the intervention using standardised instruments, scoring these measures and then undertaking statistical analyses of these scores.[95] Having SMART objectives and goals (see Chapter 12) makes analysis of the quantitative data considerably easier as the level of intended effects is clearly specified. Qualitative approaches ask 'why?' and quantitative approaches examine 'by how much?'

In the evaluation and intelligence phases both approaches are used to interpret what is happening. The extent to which each method is determined by the intervention strategies, the target group and the size of the intervention. It is most effective, however, to use a combination of qualitative and quantitative approaches.

Knowledge

Measuring knowledge involves assessing what people know, recognise, are aware of, understand and have learned. Measuring knowledge is commonly divided between measuring awareness or recognition of an intervention or intervention message and measuring what the target audiences have understood or have learnt about an issue or subject area.

Awareness of an intervention or key message is commonly used to measure social marketing and communication campaigns. This form of measurement may involve presenting representatives of the target group with a list of different campaigns/messages (a combination of real and fictitious) which includes the intervention and asking them about their awareness of each item on the list. Measuring awareness using a variety of prompts avoids the 'demand characteristic' of asking a more direct question about the intervention (e.g. 'Are you aware of a recent healthy eating campaign?'), to which most people will respond 'yes'.[89] However, an open, 'unprompted' question (e.g. 'Can you name any healthy eating campaigns you have seen in the past six months?') can be asked before offering a list of prompts. However, it is important to bear in mind when measuring knowledge that, unless they have agreed to be involved in a learning situation such as a training course, people tend not to respond positively when asked: 'What did you learn?' Most think they do not need to be taught anything.

Assessing knowledge about an intervention or subject matter can be undertaken in several ways, three of which are described below.

- *Recall* – Assessed by asking: 'What did the campaign/intervention encourage people to do?'
- *Learning* – Participants are asked to mark statements about a particular topic as true or false or select the correct response from a series of alternatives (multiple-choice format).
- *Change in knowledge* – Before and after questionnaires using a similar format as above. Take care with questionnaires which ask people to rate their knowledge of a subject as being aware of the complexity of a topic can cause people to become modest in their self-assessment post-intervention.[89]

Attitudes and self-efficacy

Measuring attitude and self-efficacy involves assessing how people feel about the intervention or topic, or their ability to participate in intervention activities, and commonly involves qualitative methods which encourage greater freedom of expression.[89] Methods of exploring attitudes include showing short films, role-plays or picture/verbal stories of scenarios depicting the topic of interest, for example, showing a family eating a takeaway meal with a soft drink while watching television and asking: 'What do you think about this family's evening meal habits and the foods they are consuming?' Responses can be collected through individual interviews, a focus group or a questionnaire (Table 17.1). Self-efficacy can be measured in a similar way by asking how the individual feels about their ability to undertake and continue intervention activities.

Table 17.1   Questionnaire for measuring attitudes

Please circle the response that most closely matches how you feel about each statement	
Eating the evening meal while watching television promotes healthy eating habits	Strongly agree Agree Don't know Disagree Strongly disagree
Eating takeaway foods five times a week is healthy	Strongly agree Agree Don't know Disagree Strongly disagree
It is healthy for families to eat the evening meal together seated at the dining table	Strongly agree Agree Don't know Disagree Strongly disagree

Source: Adapted from Hawe et al.[89]

Behaviour

The purpose of most PHN interventions is to bring about change in people's dietary and activity behaviour (i.e. to eat more nutritious foods and take more exercise). Measuring behaviour can be achieved through self-report, however this is generally not accurate because of the social desirability attached to healthy eating and engaging in regular physical activity. Asking people to record their behaviour in a food and exercise diary over time can minimise inaccuracy, however, it can also influence behaviour, making the reporting process more a part of the intervention than of the evaluation.[89]

Observation is another way to measure behaviour. Although sometimes considered inconvenient, observation may be the most effective method of measuring behaviour.[89] Observation may include watching the food choices employees or students make in a work or school canteen, asking participants to photograph their dinner plates on a specially designed placemat before eating or calculating product consumption from sales data.

Health status

When selecting an appropriate health status measure for impact or outcome evaluation it is important first to revisit the intended effect of the intervention and then to ensure the selected measure includes the necessary dimensions and is suited to the target group. In PHN interventions health status can be measured using biochemical or anthropometric indicators for diet-related conditions such as obesity, glucose intolerance, diabetes and cardiovascular disease, or measures of physical fitness.

Social support

PHN interventions may attempt to increase the quality and quantity of social support given to a target population such as young parents, newly arrived immigrants or people living in disadvantaged communities. There is a variety of self-completed questionnaires and interview schedules available to measure social support. Selecting which measure is most appropriate depends on the aspect of social support the intervention is emphasising, such as the extent to which the social support provides information, practical assistance, self-efficacy or meets the individual's expectations. Simple measures can also be used – for example, the number of young mothers who can provide the names of each other's partners or children, or if they have visited each other's homes since commencing the intervention.[89]

Environmental support

Many comprehensive PHN interventions aim to bring about change at an environmental level as well as changing social and behavioural factors. Measuring environmental support considers change in the physical environment, policies, legislation and workforce support. For example, an intervention targeting physical activity in the workplace may measure environmental support by auditing the work environment, considering the availability of secure bike racks, shower, locker or gym facilities, accessibility of stairwells and changes in organisational policy about active commuting, flexible working hours or salary packaging. Environmental audit tools for different surroundings such as schools, workplaces and communities are becoming more readily available.

Reliability and validity in evaluation

While it is not possible to detail the process of constructing the various evaluation tools outlined above (questionnaires and scales, interviews and focus groups, etc.) there are two important technical concepts to consider when developing evaluation tools to assess changes in knowledge, attitudes, behaviours and environmental or social factors; these are reliability and validity.

Reliability is the stability of a measure. A reliable tool measures the same things each time the measure is used and for each person it is used with. The most common method used to test and develop reliability is to repeat administration of the measurement on the same subject using the same administration procedures within a short period of time to ensure this 'test–retest' procedure elicits the same results.[95] If the same participant answers a set of questions in relation to a specific behaviour or nutrition problem in the same way within a relatively short period of time the measurement tool can be considered reliable. Testing for reliability is also important for observable indicators, such as observing or rating the physical activity characteristics of a community. Reliability of an observation tool can be determined by the level of agreement between two observers of the same phenomenon. This is known as 'inter-rater reliability'. If the observations differed markedly, the measurement tool is unreliable and strict guidelines need to be developed for the manner in which data are collected; alternatively, the number of observers can be limited to minimise variations in observation.[95]

Validity is the truth of a measure. A valid tool measures what it intends to measure. A common approach to assess validity is the use of biochemical or physiological tests, where these tests are considered 'true' measures of the factors of interest, for example, the measurement of blood lipids to validate aspects of self-reported diet. Although desirable, such measures are generally difficult and expensive, not always practical to use and are only available to support measures of behaviour.

Measurement of attitudes and beliefs, and psychological concepts such as self-efficacy (very important for increasing physical activity), cannot be objectively assessed, however, a simple procedure of face validity and content validity can be employed to check validity. *Face validity* involves experts in the field agreeing that the measure is a useful way of assessing the phenomenon in question. *Content validity* ensures that all the areas of the phenomenon in question are covered by measurement items[95] – for example, a valid questionnaire presents options in a balanced manner and allows respondents to answer across the full range of potential responses. By asking respondents how much they agree/disagree with a statement respondents are able to express their answer in different degrees, and the evaluator is able to analyse the difference in response in a more sophisticated, systematic manner. This question design presents potential responses in the form of a ranked scale ('strongly agree', 'agree', neither nor disagree', 'disagree', 'strongly disagree') and is called a *Likert scale*.

Valid measures of concepts such as social capital or capacity building are more challenging to develop because concepts are factors in a causal chain that are not directly observable. As a result, turning concepts into actual measures is a technical process derived from psychology and other social sciences. The aim is to turn concepts into variables that can reliably and validly show variation among subjects and variation as a consequence of intervention.[95] For example, there is no direct measure for observing community capacity, however this concept can be described and relevant questions generated, administered to the target group and psychometric statistical techniques used to describe how well the questions relate to the construct or how well the construct exists. This process helps assess *construct validity*. Techniques for measuring capacity gains are further explained in Chapter 18.

It is important to note that a reliable tool is not necessarily a valid tool, as it may be measuring the wrong thing but doing so consistently. It is also worth researching the literature for published instruments or measures before designing a new measure. Using available measures will enable a comparison with published data and save considerable time and resources.

Sampling and data analysis

Impact and outcome evaluation designs should consider potential sources of bias, sampling methods and methods of data analysis, each of which is outlined below.

Sampling bias

Bias exists where something differs systematically from the true situation and influences the evaluation conclusions. Sampling bias concerns the characteristics of intervention participants, the reasons for their participation and the duration of their participation. How participants are recruited to participate in the intervention and whether they are representative of the whole target population have an important impact on the evaluation findings. For example, those who volunteer to participate in an intervention or evaluation may have greater motivation or health literacy than those who do not volunteer and can distort the intervention results by producing better outcomes than if a more representative population participated in the intervention. It is particularly important to address this type of bias in an intervention which aims to have the greatest impact among marginalised or disadvantaged populations.

Sampling bias can also arise as a consequence of non-response, when a person appropriate to participate in the intervention declines to do so. This form of bias also produces different effects from those that would be observed if the programme were delivered to a fully representative population. For example, if an intervention was targeting 200 maternal and child health nurses in a particular region, and only 20 senior nurses participated, the evaluation data may be limited by the non-response bias associated with obtaining evaluation data from participants who do not represent the target population. The consequence of both forms of sampling bias is that the results cannot be generalised and extrapolated to the target population as a whole. Another source of sampling bias concerns subject retention. This type of bias can occur if participants who drop out of the intervention or participate in the baseline data collection only are different from those who complete the intervention and/or the follow-up data collection. The extent of drop-out or loss to follow-up can influence the usefulness and generalisability of the results.

It is important to do all that is practically possible to obtain a representative sample and maintain the participation rate throughout the intervention to avoid sampling bias. It is similarly important to collect data about the evaluation participants so that assessments about sample representativeness can be considered. Strategies to retain participants include using easy-to-complete questionnaires, ongoing communication or incentives. When analysing impact and outcome evaluation results, any sampling bias should be described and the possible influence on results outlined.

Sampling methods

Sampling methods for impact and outcome evaluation tend to differ according to the size of the PHN intervention. In small-scale interventions it may be possible to measure the intervention effect in all participants. Most PHN interventions, however, rely on a subset from the population to assess the impact and outcome of the intervention. A random sample is considered the best method for evaluating intervention effects in large population groups because the effects of the intervention can be considered to apply to the entire target population. Taking a random sample requires a list of the whole target population to be available and that it is possible to select subjects at random. Examples of population lists include censuses, employee payrolls, school registers and telephone listings. It may not always be possible or practical to achieve a true random sample. Table 17.2 illustrates different types of sampling which can be used for impact and outcome evaluation of PHN interventions.

Statistical analysis

It is essential to consider the use of statistical methods to analyse and make sense of the quantitative data collected from impact and outcome evaluation. Statistical analysis allows evaluation data to be interpreted and produces useful information about the success/failure of an intervention. Statistical methods should be taken into account during evaluation planning to determine the sample size of the evaluation and which statistical tests to apply. Key statistical considerations include:

- *Statistical significance* – The probability of the observed result occurring by chance. Often described as p values of <0.05 or <0.01, indicating there is a 1 in 20 or 1 in 100 possibility of an observed outcome by chance respectively.
- *Confidence intervals* – Describe how likely it is that the true population results are outside the range described by the confidence limits.

Table 17.2 Sampling and recruitment methods for evaluation of large and small PHN interventions

	Recruitment of participants – small PHN intervention	Sampling of participants – large PHN intervention
	A trial of a community kitchen intervention to increase healthy eating knowledge and skills with newly arrived immigrants	A national school programme to increase reduced-fat dairy intake and physical activity levels in children aged 5–12 years
Best sampling method (generalisable) ↓ Less useful sampling method (less reliable)	Random sampling from target population of newly arrived immigrants Sampling from a defined database of older people Sampling from numerous community groups and clinical settings – even if non-random may be adequately diverse to be generalisable Snowball samples where hard-to-reach groups are found through social networks – can produce reasonable samples Volunteer immigrants recruited through newspaper/newsletter advertisements	Random sample of children aged 5–12 is measured – sampling of the at-risk whole population gives every individual an equal chance of selection Other variants: Random sampling with increased samples (over-sampling) of specific groups of interest, particularly those attending schools in more disadvantaged areas Universal sampling where everyone is surveyed because the target population is small Non-random (convenient) sampling – volunteers responding to a letter sent home, local sporting clubs, selected classes

Source: Adapted from Nutbeam and Bauman.[95]

Different statistical tests are required for continuous data such as daily vegetable intake (*t*-tests and Pearson coefficients) compared to category data such as vegetable intake improved/did not improve (χ-squared statistics and odds ratios).

Practice note

The 'best' approach to PHN intervention evaluation varies according to the context and setting, the resources and time available, and the requirements for evidence of intervention effectiveness. A general rule for costing evaluation in funding submission and intervention plans is 20% of the total intervention budget. However, this level is not always available and when the budget is limited, evaluation designs tend to rely more heavily on the use of information describing the process of implementation (process evaluation) and qualitative interpretation of observed changes in the target group.

Evaluation design

While randomised control trials are considered the gold standard in health because they are seen as reliable and valid, their use in health promotion and public health interventions is limited.[98] There are a number of possible impact and outcome evaluation designs which are outlined in Table 17.3.

Table 17.3 Possible evaluation designs for PHN interventions

Design type	Description	Considerations
Single group, post-test only	A single measurement at the completion of the intervention is taken on the participants only.	Unsure whether the intervention actually had an effect and that any effect was actually caused by the intervention.
Single group, pre- and post-test	Two measurements are taken on the participants, one before and one after the intervention.	Pre-/post-design enables change to be observed, but cannot be certain that other factors caused or contributed to the effect.
Non-equivalent control group, pre- and post-test	Two measurements are taken, one before and one after, on an intervention and a control group. 'Non-equivalent' means the two groups are not exactly matched in characteristics and may be from another region, time period, etc.	Pre-/post-design enables change to be observed; however, because the groups are not matched it may be group differences rather than the intervention which cause the effect. It is possible to statistically control for known differences.
Single group, time-series	Multiple measures over a period of time on participants only.	Able to observe natural changes occurring in the participant group, and the size and direction of these and changes before implementing the intervention and then observe the effects. Important to consider possible external influences during the time period.
Non-equivalent, time-series	Multiple measures over a period of time on an intervention and a non-equivalent, control group.	Stronger evidence than the previous design because it more definitely rules out external factors and helps to cancel secular trends that can be missed with pre-/post-designs.
Randomised control trial	Two measurements are taken, one before and one after, on an intervention and an equivalent control group.	Overcomes all issues of the other designs.

Source: Adapted from Nutbeam and Bauman[95] and Thorogood and Coombs.[98]

Selecting an evaluation design for an intervention depends on the context, particularly the financial and staffing resources and the baseline data. Although some designs are considered more scientifically sound than others because they elicit stronger evidence about intervention effects, some are easier to execute; hence design selection is about finding the balance best suited to the context.

Key points

- Impact and outcome evaluation involve measuring the effects of an intervention, investigating the direction and degree of change and testing the proposed causal change or logic model of the population nutrition problem.
- Impact evaluation is concerned with the assessment of the immediate effects of the intervention and usually corresponds with the measurement of the intervention objective. Outcome evaluation is concerned with measuring the longer-term effects of the intervention which usually corresponds to the intervention goal.
- Predicting when the intervention effect(s) will take place and the timing of impact and outcome evaluation are very important because measuring effects too early or too late will deliver misleading findings about the intervention's effectiveness.
- Common measures used in impact and outcome evaluation in PHN interventions include knowledge, attitude and self-efficacy, behaviour, health status, social support and environmental support. A mix of qualitative and quantitative methods is used, and where possible these measures should be reliable and valid.

Chapter 18

Step 15: Evaluating capacity gains

Objectives

On completion of this chapter, you should be able to:

1. Evaluate capacity gains using a multi-modular framework for capacity evaluation.
2. Descriptively summarise and justify assessments of capacity gain using examples and evidence.
3. Use visual representations of capacity evaluation data to illustrate effectiveness of capacity building strategies.

Practical Public Health Nutrition, first edition. Roger Hughes and Barrie M. Margetts. Published 2011 by Blackwell Publishing Ltd. © 2011 Roger Hughes and Barrie M. Margetts.

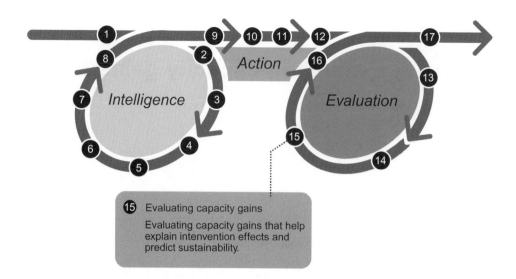

Introduction

Earlier chapters have emphasised the critical importance of a capacity building approach to PHN practice. Capacity building is a strategy and capacity gain is an outcome. Capacity building as a strategy needs to be evaluated so that judgements can be made about the effectiveness of capacity building strategies. Given the critical importance of capacity (the ability to achieve stated goals and objectives) in effective strategy implementation, evaluation of capacity gain is too important to ignore. Surprisingly, it has been a much neglected aspect of PHN practice – in fact, of most health promotion practice. This chapter revisits capacity assessment first considered in Chapter 8) and details how to assess capacity gains, justify and describe the intelligence used to make assessments and visually represent these data.

Challenges in measuring capacity

Building capacity to implement community-based interventions effectively is an integral part of 'doing' public health nutrition. This 'doing' focus is integrally linked to and dependent on measuring capacity.

Capacity assessment serves to:

- identify a communities readiness for action;
- engage the community;
- focus strategies for capacity building;
- provide baseline data for capacity building evaluation.

Assessment of capacity is required at various stages of capacity development and different measures may be necessary at each stage. Initial assessment of capacity provides the context for capacity building and identifies capacity building possibilities and gaps. Progressive assessments monitor change in capacity at individual, organisational and systematic levels. Impact measurement assesses the amount of capacity gain at the various levels, as well as the successful elements of the capacity building strategy and their contribution to the intervention outcomes.

The method of measuring baseline capacity, changes in capacity and the benefits of capacity building to health can be challenging and a number of issues influencing measurement of capacity have been identified from the Canadian health promotion capacity building experience.[99] These issues are not mutually exclusive – many of them interact with each other – and are not that different from measurement issues in other areas of research and evaluation. The key issues and challenges in measuring capacity are our outlined in Table 18.1.

A number of strategies to address the identified issues in measuring capacity have been suggested based on health promotion capacity research in Canada.[99] Implementing these strategies showed that a single strategy could address more than one of the measurement issues, and that a single measurement issue could be addressed by several strategies.

The strategies to address issues in measuring capacity, and the measurement issues that strategy can address are presented in Table 18.2.

Table 18.1   Issues in measuring capacity relevant to PHN interventions

Issues	Description
Multiple understandings of terms	Lack of consistent understanding of health promotion terminology across settings, organisations and individuals presents a measurement challenge as common terminology cannot be assumed when exploring health promotion capacity with key informants at multiple levels of an organisation or across sectors. This issue has implications in the design and format of measurement tools and for data analysis.
Evolving understanding of capacity	The definition and nature of capacity are evolving, so measurement tools – particularly quantitative tools – can be lengthy and complex in order to tap into the actual or potential dimensions. Respondent burden becomes an issue.
Invisibility of capacity building	Community empowerment is explicit in health promotion, which often creates a culture of invisibility around capacity building (i.e. *because capacity building practitioners want the community to take ownership and credit for capacity gains and the associated outcomes, they may not overtly communicate or promote capacity building strategies*). Invisibility causes difficulty in recognising, describing and measuring capacity building.
Dynamic contexts	The health system is dynamic and always seems to be threatening dramatic restructuring. Prominent contextual aspects that have influenced the measurement of capacity include: staff turnover, health system renewal, conflicting perspectives across informants within organisations, conflicting personalities within organisations and between informants and practitioners, 'turf' protection by health workers in different departments and organisational staff understanding and valuing the capacity building process.
Time course for change	The long-term outcome is that enhanced capacity will ultimately contribute to improved health in the population. Organisational and/ or individual capacity serve as an intermediate outcome, as do enhanced health promotion and prevention skills, services and programmes. The time course for such individual or system changes to occur is a challenge for projects with set time-frames.
Building trust and dealing with sensitive issues	It is important to develop a trusting relationship between practitioners and organisational or community representatives to ensure high-quality data collection. Equally important is the longitudinal nature of the research which requires multiple connections over time. The relationships underlying these connections depend on trust and are a mediating factor that should not be underestimated. The development of appropriate questions and the documenting and sharing of such sensitive information without breaching confidentiality or trust pose a measurement challenge.
Snapshot measurements	Quantitative instruments provide a snapshot in time. Qualitative interviews allow the exploration of critical events, milestones or snapshots, however they rely on accurate and comprehensive recall of informants, sometimes months after a particular occurrence. This can be a limitation owing to recall bias.

Table 18.1 *Continued*

Issues	Description
Validity and reliability of quantitative measures	There is no gold standard to measure health promotion capacity. Establishing criterion validity is therefore compromised. External validity, the generalisability of findings to and across populations and settings, is difficult because each project is context-specific.
Attribution for change in capacity	The process for building health promotion capacity is participatory in that organisations and individuals who are the recipients of the capacity-building interventions are integrally involved in developing, planning and evaluating the process. If the principles of participatory action and health promotion are followed, then 'others' take ownership and embrace the work as their own. This is both a positive aspect of the process and an outcome. However, identifying both the successful elements of the capacity building strategy and the independent contributions of the intervention becomes complex.

Source: Adapted from Gibbon et al.[99]

Table 18.2 Strategies to address key capacity measurement issues

Strategy	Measurement issue addressed
Utilise participatory processes as intervention	Multiple understandings of terms Evolving understanding of capacity Building trust and dealing with sensitive issues
Acknowledge the context	Invisibility of capacity building Dynamic context
Incorporate mixed methods (qualitative and quantitative)	Invisibility of capacity building Dynamic contexts Time course for change Building trust and dealing with sensitive issues Snapshot measures Validity and reliability of quantitative methods Attribution for change in capacity
Build on previous phases of community and stakeholder engagement	Multiple understandings of terms Building trust and dealing with sensitive issues
Establish validity of quantitative measures	Validity and reliability of quantitative methods
Establish trustworthiness of qualitative intelligence	Multiple understanding of terms Evolving understanding of capacity Time course for change Building trust and dealing with sensitive issues Snapshot measures
Be flexible and adaptable	Dynamic contexts Multiple understanding of terms Building trust and dealing with sensitive issues
Identify intervention contributions (i.e. intervention-specific evaluations)	Attribution for change in capacity

Source: Adapted from Gibbon et al.[99]

Practice note

In response to and guided by these challenges, a checklist for capacity assessment and evaluation has been developed based on a framework for capacity building developed by Baillie et al.[52] This can be used as a basis for developing a process for assessing and evaluating capacity gains relative to individual interventions in different contexts.

Pre- and post-intervention comparisons

Capacity assessment before capacity building strategies and activities are implemented provides a baseline for capacity gain evaluation. Pre- and post-intervention evaluation designs (time-series designs) are most commonly used in evaluation because they are simple and logical. (Figure 18.1). The weakness in this approach relates to attribution of causation (i.e. the strategies caused capacity gains rather than some other confounding factor, which provides an alternative explanation of why change has been observed). It may be possible to consider evaluating capacity gains in a sub-population or setting that receives the capacity building strategies and comparing capacity with a similar (control) population that gets usual or no strategy implementation. (Figure 18.2). Comparing the capacity assessment scores between each population or setting may provide stronger evidence that the interventions are the explanation for gains in capacity as assessed after the intervention.

Practice note

Given the current state of subjectivity associated with capacity assessment and evaluation methods, it may seem pedantic to be concerned with confounding when more relevant questions remain such as measurement validity and bias. In this case, transparency is the key, making explicit ratings and discussing observable changes that reflect capacity gains.

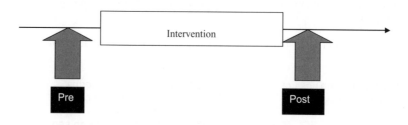

Capacity Gain = Post CBA scores - Pre CBA scores

Cannot differentiate real gains from confounding (alternative) causes

Figure 18.1   Uncontrolled pre-/post-comparisons

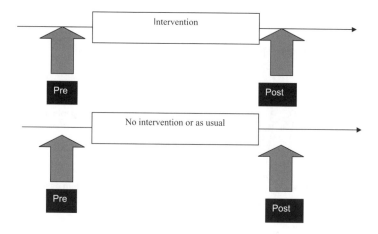

Capacity gain = Intervention (post-CBA scores − pre-CBA scores) compared to control (post-CBA scores − pre CBA scores)

Figure 18.2   Comparison with a control

Strategies to enhance the trustworthiness of capacity evaluation

Transparency

The capacity assessment tool developed by Baillie et al.[52] provides a space for the evaluator to describe changes in capacity by each capacity element/question. This enables evaluators to make explicit and transparent the changes that justify the changes in ratings noted.

Mixed-method evaluation and data triangulation

In Chapter 8, we stated that measurement of capacity and the effects of capacity building efforts can be difficult to quantify and that mixed-method approaches are required. Mixed-method approaches, such as focus groups, interviews, questionnaires and objective measures of behaviour exploring similar evaluation questions, can provide evidence of change via data triangulation. (Triangulation is an analytical strategy to identify consistencies in data from different methods, and is commonly used in qualitative research and evaluation.)

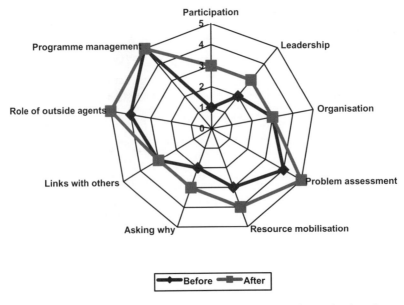

Figure 18.3 Example visual a spider's web representation to assist evaluation of community building
Source: Adapted from Bjaras et al.[100]

Visual presentations of capacity evaluations

The 'spider's web' developed by Bjaras et al.[100] (Figure 18.3) and used by others has been used to measure community participation in Sweden. The principle can be applied to demonstrate change in capacity as a response to capacity building strategies in a time-series design.

The spider's web visual enables evaluators and the communities they are working with to decide how many domains they will rate or score against and to define a system for scoring. Time-delineated points of assessment are used (e.g. before vs. after) to map change in scores in each domain.

Assessment can be either:

- *Internal* – Self-assessed by communities or partners.
- *External* – Assessed by evaluators from the available evidence (which may include data from interviews with community members, etc.).

In Table 18.3 eight community capacity domains are described and provide examples of the domains of community capacity that might be used.

Table 18.3   Capacity building domains

Domain	Description
Participation	Participation is basic to community empowerment. Only by participating in small groups or larger organisations can individual community members better define, analyse and act on issues of general concern to the broader community.
Leadership	Participation and leadership are closely connected. Leadership requires a strong participant base just as participation requires the direction and structure of strong leadership. Both play an important role in the development of small groups and community organisations.
Organisational structures	Organisational structures in a community include small groups such as committees, and church and youth groups. These are the organisational elements which represent the ways in which people come together in order to socialise and address their concerns and problems. The existence of and the level at which these organisations function is crucial to community empowerment.
Problem assessment	Empowerment presumes that the identification of problems, solutions to the problems and actions to resolve the problems are carried out by the community. This process assists communities to develop a sense of self-determination and capacity.
Resource mobilisation	The ability of the community to mobilise resources from within and to negotiate resources from beyond itself is important to its ability so achieve successes in its efforts.
Asking why	The ability of the community to critically assess the social, political, economic and other causes of inequalities is a crucial stage towards developing appropriate personal and social change strategies.
Links with others	Links with people and organisations, including partnerships, coalitions and voluntary alliances between the community and others, can assist the community to address its issues.
Role of the outside agents	In a programme context, outside agents are often an important link between communities and external resources. Their role is especially important near the beginning of a new programme, when the process of building new community momentum may be triggered and nurtured. The outside agent increasingly transforms power relationships between her/himself, outside agencies and the community, such that the community assumes increasing programme authority.
Programme management	Programme management that empowers the community includes the control by the primary stakeholders over decisions on planning, implementation, evaluation, finances, administration, reporting and conflict resolution. The first step towards programme management by the community is to define the roles, responsibilities and line management of all the stakeholders.

Source: Adapted from Gibbon et al.[99]

Key points

- Evaluating capacity gain is an important step in PHN intervention practice; however, there are currently limited tools to support quantitative evaluation.
- Practitioners need to apply mixed-method approaches to collect intelligence about capacity gains, and be flexible and context-specific in these assessments.

Chapter 19

Step 16: Economic evaluation

Objectives

On completion of this chapter, students should be able to:

1. Describe the value of economic evaluation in PHN intervention management.
2. Identify and detail the different types of economic evaluation.
3. Apply an economic evaluation framework to PHN interventions to measure intervention efficiency
4. Explain the relationship between effectiveness, efficiency and equity in economic evaluation.

Practical Public Health Nutrition, first edition. Roger Hughes and Barrie M. Margetts. Published 2011 by Blackwell Publishing Ltd. © 2011 Roger Hughes and Barrie M. Margetts.

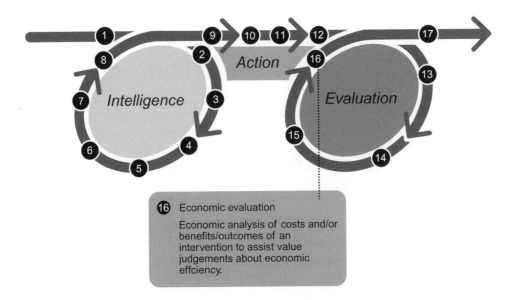

16 Economic evaluation

Economic analysis of costs and/or benefits/outcomes of an intervention to assist value judgements about economic effciency.

Introduction

Economic evaluation is an underused but arguably essential component of PHN intervention evaluation. Economic evaluation considers assessment of intervention effects in economic terms, which is often of great interest to fund allocators. Economic evaluation requires considerable expertise, which is often outside the scope of an individual public health nutritionist's competence. It is, though, important to consider economic evaluation opportunities in the context of evaluation planning and practice.

Costs and consequences in health care

Economic evaluation is an essential component of PHN intervention evaluation. Intervention evaluation involves two measures: (a) the health effects or effectiveness of the intervention (impact, outcome and capacity gain measures); and (b) the value or efficiency of the effects (economic evaluation). Knowing the outcomes or effects of an intervention is essential for economic evaluation to be undertaken; no intervention can be more efficient or cost-effective than the alternatives unless it is effective.[101] Performing economic evaluation of PHN interventions is important to enable comparisons between interventions with similar and different outcomes and help decision-makers prioritise society's scarce health care resources.[102]

In a truly practical sense, economics is the ultimate arbiter of intervention implementation. Resources for public health nutrition and health promotion are finite, so ensuring value for money is an important objective for those delivering and funding interventions.[103,104] Professionals in preventive health practice should not underestimate the importance of the costs and consequences of the activities they deliver. Health funding is limited and prevention activities are notoriously under-funded owing to political power residing in the traditional medicine disciplines and a tendency to overplay the role of treating illness rather than preparing the well for continuing health. Economic evaluations can show comparisons of public health and health promotion interventions in terms of the value of treatment interventions.[105]

Characteristics of economic evaluation

Economic evaluation involves identifying, measuring and valuing the inputs (costs) and outcomes (benefits) of the intervention(s) and their selection is determined by the problem being addressed and the perspective of the study. As discussed in Chapter 14, the intervention goal and objectives set the criteria of success for the intervention outcomes according to the determinant analysis of the PHN problem.

In terms of perspective, there are two broad areas for economic measurement:

1 *Provider or narrow perspective* – The evaluation is designed for a particular customer, commonly the organisation implementing or funding the intervention, who needs to understand the costs involved, the potential savings resulting from the intervention and what improvements in health the target population will gain.

Table 19.1   Characteristics of partial and full economic evaluations

		Are both costs and benefits analysed?		
		NO		**YES**
Is there comparison of two or more alternatives?	No	Examines only consequences	Examines only costs	
		Outcome description	**Cost description**	**Cost outcome description**
	Yes	Effectiveness evaluation	Cost analysis	Full economic evaluation • Cost-minimisation analysis • Cost-effectiveness analysis • Cost-utility analysis • Cost-benefit analysis

2   *Societal perspective* – Evaluation involves considering a broader impact than that immediately affecting the provider, to capture all relevant costs borne by the provider and the benefits accruing to potential beneficiaries, to produce an aggregate of all costs and benefits across society as a whole.[105]

Economists would argue that the provider approach has great limitations because the ranking of interventions in terms of value for money may be very different if the analysis includes all costs and benefits, and not just those incurred by the provider.

A further distinction can be made between evaluations of health interventions *Full evaluations* consider inputs (costs) and outcomes (benefits), and compare both aspects across alternative interventions. *Partial evaluations* include only some elements of inputs and outcomes.[103] Table 19.1 shows the characteristics of both types of evaluation. These characteristics are described in further detail in the next section.

Types of economic evaluation

Various types of partial evaluation include outcome description, cost analysis and/or cost outcome description and each type of measurement can be undertaken on a single intervention. Costing health promotion interventions, however, presents several problems. Many interventions involve time and resources from a range of individuals and agencies which are often engaged in numerous activities in addition to the intervention of interest. Tracing all inputs and finding valuations for all the various resources used can be very difficult in PHN interventions; however, this should not deter informed estimates being made.

A *cost outcome description* may examine, for example, the relationship between the level of resources and intervention participation. Costs in terms of resources used could be assessed by considering the community's contribution in time, money or materials, plus the professional input, including time, education materials, media costs, etc., and may be collected from questionnaires and reviewing records or receipts.[103]

Table 19.2   Different types of full economic evaluation

Type	Cost measure	Outcome identifier	Outcome measure	Comparison
Cost-minimisation analysis	Monetary terms	Identical in all respects	None	Lowest cost for equal result
Cost-effectiveness analysis	Monetary terms	Single effect of interest, common to both alternatives, but achieved to different degrees	Natural units (body weight, fruit and vegetable intake, glucose level, blood pressure, life years)	Example: $: kg lost
Cost-utility analysis	Monetary terms	Simple or multiple effects, not necessarily common to both alternatives	Quality adjusted life years (QALYs) Disability adjusted life years (DALYs)	Example: $: QALY
Cost-benefit analysis	Monetary terms	Single or multiple effects, not necessarily common to both alternatives	Monetary terms	Example: $: $

Outcome description or *effectiveness evaluation* has limited use economically, as the resources used to achieve the different outcomes are not considered. Similarly, conducting only a *cost description* or *cost analysis* is limited by the fact that economically efficient interventions do not necessarily yield the best outcomes.

Evaluations that consider both outcomes and resources can be considered full economic evaluations, of which there are four types: cost-minimisation, cost-effectiveness, cost-utility and cost-benefit. Each type expresses inputs or costs in monetary units, but are different in how the principal outcome is measured. Table 19.2 illustrates the main features of each type of full economic evaluation.

Cost-minimisation analysis

Cost-minimisation involves a comparison between two or more interventions whose outcomes are assumed to be identical. A strong assumption here is that all consequences of the alternative interventions are the same. For example, in addition to direct benefits, some PHN interventions may have consequences or additional benefits such as reducing future demands on health care resources. The individual benefits may be assumed to be the same, however interventions could have a number of further consequences, so assuming equality of all consequences in monetary terms may be difficult. Generally, this method is not recommended.[103]

Cost-effectiveness analysis

Cost-effectiveness is the most common type of economic evaluation in health care. The individual benefit is usually measured as a quantifiable unit, either behavioural (fruit and vegetable intake) or a health outcome (glucose/ blood pressure level). These measures have been criticised for failing to recognise the broader potential benefits from PHN interventions, but quantification of measures is required. Robroek et al.[106] considered the direct costs of medical service consumption (contacts with health professionals) and the indirect costs of loss of productivity in a two-year worksite health promotion programme on physical activity and nutrition in the Netherlands. The cost-effectiveness ratio was also calculated on general health and risk for cardiovascular events.

It is important to note that without a common health measure, cost-effectiveness analysis cannot be used to compare interventions. Cost-effectiveness analysis is most suitable when programmes with the same health aims are being compared and these health objectives are the primary outcomes of interest.[103]

Cost-utility analysis

Cost-utility analysis uses a common measure of outcome to enable a comparison between a range of interventions, including between health promotion interventions or between a health promotion intervention and a treatment approach.[104] Benefits or outcome measures are expressed as a measure that reflects how individuals value or gain utility from the quality and length of life, namely QALYs (quality adjusted life years), DALYS (disability adjusted life years) or HYE (health year equivalents). Calculating QALYs involves combining life expectancy with the measure of health-related quality of life attributable to the intervention. For example, if health-related quality of life is valued on a scale of 0 (death) to 1 (perfect health) and an intervention increases the quality of life for an individual from 0.5 to 0.9 for 10 years, then the intervention yields a health gain of 4 QALYs ($10 \times [0.9 - 0.5]$).

Gusi et al.[107] describe how using QALYs to assess the cost-effectiveness of adding a supervised walking programme to best practice for overweight, moderately obese and moderately depressed women in Spain. Outcome measures for the study were health care costs and QALYs. Each QALY gained by the intervention was costed against the control and was shown to be both feasible and cost-effective.

While useful for comparing outcomes across health care interventions, cost-utility measures when improvements in population health are observed but individual change is relatively small is difficult to quantify. In addition, PHN interventions can have non-health benefits for target populations, such as increasing self-efficacy or confidence, which may translate into healthier choices but not necessarily changes in health-related quality of life.[103]

Cost-benefit analysis

Cost-benefit analysis measures all outcomes in monetary terms and relies on creating or calculating the monetary value of health benefits and costs to conclude if one side is greater than the other – this is commonly expressed as a cost-benefit ratio.[105] This method is useful for comparing interventions with many diverse outcomes and is the most appropriate method for economic evaluation of inter-sectoral interventions which involve communities and numerous agencies. Utility-based health measures currently available are unlikely to capture all these outcomes.[103]

Wang et al.[108] provide an example of a cost-benefit analysis of a school-based obesity prevention programme in the USA. The costs measured were: intervention costs; medical care costs associated with adulthood overweight; and costs of productivity loss associated with adulthood overweight. The results showed that at an intervention cost of $33,677 ($14 per student per year) would prevent an estimated 1.9% of the female students becoming overweight adults. Furthermore, society could expect to save an estimated $15,887 in medical care costs and $25,104 in loss of productivity costs.

Practice note

Conducting a thorough economic evaluation required specialised health economics expertise and can be a resource-intensive process. Ideally, economic evaluation should only be undertaken if the benefits of improving efficiency of health resources outweigh the costs of evaluation.

There is no consensus on which method is best and the decision is likely to be limited to the type and quantity of information available and the time and resource restraints. *Choose a method that is most appropriate to the data available.* Although funding agencies financing PHN interventions will be interested in the economic benefit from an organisational perspective, most agencies would prefer to promote the societal benefits the intervention they funded had, hence taking a societal perspective to economic evaluation is preferred.

Conducting an economic evaluation

The main steps to consider when conducting an economic evaluation are outlined in Table 19.3. To undertake a high-quality economic evaluation a multidisciplinary team comprising economists and public health nutritionists is required. Further information about conducting an economic evaluation can be found in the reading list at the end of this chapter.

Efficiency vs. equity

It is often assumed that there is a trade-off between maximising aggregate benefits and attaining an equitable distribution across the whole population.[105] A principal criterion

Table 19.3   Main steps of economic evaluation

Step	Description
Defining the economic question and perspective	Choice of study: • Comparison between *single health promotion intervention strategies* (healthy eating social marketing vs. policy change at workplaces), or • Vomparison between *multiple health promotion intervention strategies* (social marketing and education vs. policy change plus social marketing at workplaces), or • Comparison between *health promotion and treatment alternative.* Decision to take a narrow/provider perspective or a societal perspective.
Determining the alternatives to be evaluated	Full economic evaluations require two or more alternatives to be compared. A prior appraisal reviewing costs and benefits in broad terms may help create a shortlist of options. One option is to do nothing, with a comparison between benefits and costs of the PHN intervention compared with the predicted population health/ healthcare costs of maintaining the status quo. Multi-component interventions may also be compared by comparing the results of adding different components to core activities or more intense activities with certain groups.
Choosing the evaluation design	Choosing evaluation design involves selecting the economic evaluation method (partial or full) and type. The appropriateness of choice depends on the context and PHN problem being addressed. Full economic evaluations occur at the end of the evaluation process measuring intervention progress and effectiveness. Economic data would be collected concurrently with the effectiveness data, though costs may be collated retrospectively.
Identifying, measuring and valuing the costs	The full range of costs to be identified include: • *direct costs incurred by the health promotion agency* – consumables, staff costs, overheads; • *direct costs to other agencies* – staff time, resources (other agencies will have staff and resource opportunity costs); • *direct costs to participants* – travel, childcare, other expenses including difficult-to-measure costs such as distress, worried-well syndrome; • *productivity costs* – loss of productivity due to participation during working hours, leisure time, etc. It is advisable to show these costs separately so readers can examine the estimated costing for each item. Excluding certain costs (e.g. identical costs for some items between alternatives) should be justified.

Table 19.3 *Continued*

Step	Description
Identifying, measuring and valuing the benefits	Measuring, identifying and valuing the effects of alternatives vary with each type of economic evaluation: • *cost-effectiveness analysis* – uses process measures (e.g. number of leaflets distributed) and/or outcome measures (process measures must be adequate proxies for the outcomes of the alternative intervention being compared); • *cost-utility analysis* – uses a broad health measure such as QALY or DALY (QALYs are a set of health descriptors that measure changes in health status as a result of the intervention, for example EQ-5D); • *cost-benefit analysis* – values health outcomes in monetary terms. Methodologies range from market valuations to asking people about their willingness to pay (more useful at capturing more subtle changes and can include benefits in addition to direct health benefit such as non-health benefits, social diffusion effects and effects on future resource use).
Adjusting costs and benefits for the differential timing	Some health benefits and health care savings will occur later than the direct costs of the health promotion intervention. Considering the costs and benefits over as long a period as is practicable and discounting future costs against those in the present compensates for the fact that people value future benefits or costs less than those that occur at present. This is called time discounting and is common commercial economic practice. There is much debate about the exact value and necessity of discounting in economic evaluation of health promotion interventions, particularly as discounting gives lower weight to potential future health care savings.
Measuring incremental costs and benefits	Knowing the additional costs or benefits for one extra unit of activity is an important element in economic evaluation as comparing alternatives may be more a decision between how much of A and how much of B than a choice between A and B. For example, a mass media campaign about eating fruit and vegetables may be less effective than a direct mailing strategy at low levels of expenditure, but have much greater reach and effectiveness at high levels of expenditure. Valuing the costs or benefits of units of activity may be hard to define and the average cost of a unit may vary with the level of fixed costs. For example, the set-up costs of producing 1,000 leaflets for a campaign involves all design and preparatory costs, whereas printing an extra 300 leaflets may cost only a little more.

Table 19.3 *Continued*

Step	Description
Putting the costs and benefits together	Once all the costs and benefits have been measured, valued and discounted to present values, the results can be collated. Analysis may show a clear alternative that has greater effects and lower costs, or may show that one alternative has greater effects and higher costs. Marginal analysis can ascertain the amount of extra benefit for each increase in resources available. Cost-effectiveness results should be shown as the net costs per main effect, and cost-benefit results should show the net social worth (benefit minus cost) for each unit if of the intervention compared to the alternative.
Testing the sensitivity of the results	Economic evaluations usually involve estimates of future health gains. These health gains involve uncertainties, so the sensitivities of any economic evaluation results should be tested by using different estimates of gains. Uncertainty tests can be done by using statistical properties of the estimated effects such as confidence intervals around the estimate and/or varying discounts rates.
Presenting the results	Economic evaluation is a powerful tool that can influence policy and the funding decisions of key opinion leaders. The results of economic evaluation will be useful only when presented with clarity and transparency, and address aspects of interest. It is important to avoid inappropriate generalisations.

Source: Adapted from Godfrey[103] and Stevens.[105]

for economic evaluation of maximising outcomes within a defined budget fails to account for who receives these outcomes. For example, the most cost-effective intervention may be the one directed at currently healthy, well-educated, wealthier individuals and so could result in widening health inequalities.[103]

The evaluation of an intervention is best explored in terms of effectiveness, efficiency and equity. Efficiency is the relative effectiveness of an intervention and considers resource allocation, marginal costs and the benefits to society as a whole, but does not attempt to identify which individuals or communities gain or lose.[104] Therefore, equity aims should sit alongside economic efficiency or value-for-money objectives to ensure all three dimensions of evaluation are considered. Targeting coverage rather than output can increase equity, particularly when those not reached are most likely to benefit, commonly the more disadvantaged groups – unemployed, lower education levels, lower income levels, etc.[103]

Another ethical consideration in economic evaluation is the value given to life and the comparison of worth over different individuals. Measures based on expected earnings are biased towards people with higher earning capacity and, generally, measures based on earning capacity unless when a population average is applied are not recommended. Other measures, such as QALYs, have an in-built equity component because the same worth is applied regardless of the individual.[103]

Key points

- Intervention evaluation involves two measures: (a) the health effects or effectiveness of the intervention (impact, outcome and capacity gain measures), and (b) the value or efficiency of the effects (economic evaluation).
- Performing economic evaluation of PHN interventions is important to enable comparisons between interventions with similar and different outcomes to be made and help decision-makers prioritise scarce health care resources. Economic evaluations can compare public health and health promotion interventions with treatment interventions in terms of value.
- Economic evaluations involve identifying, measuring and valuing both the inputs (costs) and outcomes (benefits) of the intervention(s); their selection is dependent on the problem being addressed and the perspective of the study. Economic measurement can have a narrow/provider perspective or a societal perspective.
- Evaluations of health interventions can be partial or full. Full evaluations consider both inputs (costs) and outcomes (benefits) and compare both aspects across alternative interventions, while partial evaluations include only some elements of inputs and outcomes. There are four distinct types of full economic evaluation: cost-minimisation, cost-effectiveness, cost-utility and cost-benefit.

Chapter 20

Step 17: Reflective practice and valorisation

Objectives

On completion of this chapter, you should be able to:

1. Describe the importance of reflective practice in PHN intervention management.
2. Apply a reflective practice framework to PHN interventions to measure intervention efficiency.
3. Identify and apply the tools and processes for valorisation of PHN intervention outcomes.

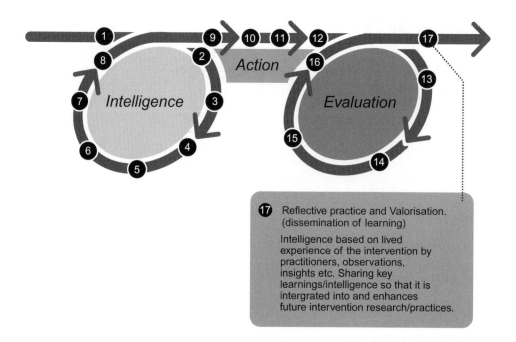

17 Reflective practice and Valorisation. (dissemination of learning)

Intelligence based on lived experience of the intervention by practitioners, observations, insights etc. Sharing key learnings/intelligence so that it is intergrated into and enhances future intervention research/practices.

Introduction

Evaluation and competent practice involve reflecting on what you have done or are doing as part of the professional learning process. At the end of the PHN intervention management bi-cycle the PHN practitioner should be looking ahead with the wealth of experience that looking back has provided. Reflective practice prompts self-evaluation, which improves and adds to the quality of the activity undertaken.

What is reflective practice?

Reflective practice is an ongoing process involving thoughtful consideration of one's own experiences to learn from and enhance practice. In 1983, Donald Schön[109] suggested that the capacity to 'reflect on action' is to engage in a process of continuous learning and was one of the defining characteristics of professional practice. Reflection on action occurs after the encounter or after an activity has been completed and may involve a practitioner writing records or a journal about the encounter or discussing it with a colleague or supervisor. The act of reflecting on action enables practitioners to spend time exploring why they acted as they did, what occurred in the group, what the response of participants and stakeholders was, and so on. Reflection develops a set of questions and ideas about the professional's activities and practice from which to learn and improve future activity and practice.[110] In this way, reflective practice becomes a source of intelligence that is as useful as objective intelligence and feeds into the continuation of the PHN intervention management bi-cycle into the next intelligence stage.

Reflection is about exploration and demands rigour, self-discipline and self-critique. Reflecting on one's own practice provides autonomy to interpret events personally experienced. Freedom in experiential learning can bring about self-transformatory learning, but will only take place if the insight gained is acted on and the change is valued.[111]

Transformatory learning and reflective practice

Transformatory learning explains how our culturally framed assumptions and presuppositions become concepts within which we operate and which give meaning to our experiences and professional practice. Reflection can enable the practitioner to challenge previous ways of thinking, and may come to see the world differently and in turn come to act differently.[112] Reflective practice and transformatory learning are particularly important when working with new population groups, a range of stakeholders and engaging in capacity building strategies where prior assumptions or expectations can be challenged or reconsidered.

Improving practice through reflection

Reflective practice is an essential element of professional development and expert practice. Competent practitioners are those actively involved in constructing and reconstructing concepts of good practice during and after the course of professional action. Expert practitioners are those with 'conscious expertise', who are willing to reflect and learn from experience, and are open-minded and do not function in isolation.[112] Self-evaluation through reflection creates self-awareness and intellectual growth and develops an understanding of what constitutes good practice and one's own level of ability.

Reflective practice can be considered a companion or precursor to professional development by assessing the congruency of practice behaviour with personal/professional values and beliefs, and assisting autonomous practice through self-monitoring and accountability.[112] Reflective practice has been explicitly linked with the development of competent practice and prevention of complacency on practice.

Stages of reflective practice

Reflective practice requires the practitioner to engage actively in examining themselves, themselves in relation to others and themselves in relation to their context. This form of reflection requires considerable self-monitoring and discipline, but encourages autonomy by facilitating the ability to monitor one's own development.[112] The process of reflection involves progressing through three key stages which are briefly outlined with an example in Table 20.1.

Methods of reflective practice

Critical reflection is a developmental process because the ability to recognise, accept and value one's own thinking often takes time and practice.[6] While reflection may be a natural part of personal growth for some practitioners, for others becoming a reflective practitioner requires motivation and support. There are various methods employed to perform reflective practice. These can be applied according to personal preference, reflective experience and the situation or context on which the reflection is based. Descriptions of the key reflective methods are provided in Table 20.2.

Research suggests that open-ended reflective journals encourage critical reflection and promote insight, self-development and an approach for life-long learning. However, journaling may be perceived as a difficult, time-consuming and continuous exercise requiring much effort, particularly when there is competing commitments.[113]

The critique/mentoring method is considered a motivational process because in a supportive environment professionals are encouraged to revisit their reflective writings, to offer justifications for positions taken and respond to open-ended questions and alternatives. As a result practitioners develop confidence in reflection and critical thinking skills.[113] Practitioners are encouraged to apply a combination of reflective practice methods because the methods are complementary and can further enhance practice when used together. Table 20.3 shows a model of reflection for practice development which highlights where each reflective practice method is generally applied.

Table 20.1   Stages of reflection

Stage	Description	Example
1	Awareness of uncomfortable feelings and thoughts • Experience of surprise • Inner discontent • Affective, discriminant, judgemental reflectivity	A very unproductive intervention management committee meeting has left you feeling frustrated and surprised about the lack of agreement on intervention strategies, particularly the slogan and design of the social marketing strategy.
2	Critical analysis of the situation • Reflection and criticism • Openness to new information and perspectives • Resolution • Conceptual, psychic and theoretical reflectivity • Association, integration, validation and appropriation	You describe a reflection about the meeting and how it makes you feel. You then share and discuss the writing with a trusted colleague to question and critique your reflection and assist you in considering the situation and your role more rationally.
3	Development of new perspective • Establishing continuity of self with past, present and future • Deciding whether and how to take action • Perspective transformation • Cognitive, affective and behavioural changes • Action	You decide on an appropriate course of action for future meetings and how you will present options and how you will react to criticism and approach disagreement among the key stakeholders.

Source: Adapted from Freshwater.[112]

Table 20.2   Methods for reflective practice

Method	Descriptions
Reflective journaling	Regularly scribed narratives and analysis of practice and professional experiences. Can enable the development of awareness and provide the opportunity to highlight habitual thinking.
Reflective writing	Any form of writing that can be used to assist with learning from experience.
Critique/feedback	Non-judgemental feedback/questioning given by a supervisor or colleague on a professional's practice or reflective writing in an effort to promote further development of self-awareness and logical reasoning skills.
Mentoring	Formalised relationship between colleagues where the more senior colleague supports critical, innovative and explorative thinking through questioning and providing feedback to enhance professional practice and competence.

Source: Adapted from Freshwater.[112]

Table 20.3 Model of reflection for practice development

Level of reflection	Method of reflection	Stages of development
Descriptive	Reflective journal Reflective writings	Practice becomes conscious

Dialogic	Discussion with peers in
	  various arenas, including
	  supervisors or managers
	  (feedback)
		Practice becomes
		  deliberate

Critical	Ability to provide reasoning
	  for actions by engaging
	  in critical conversation
	  with mentor/self/others
		Transformation of
		  practice
		Practice development
		Innovation

Source: Adapted from Freshwater.[112]

Tools for reflective practice

Two tools can be of use to a reflective PHN practitioner. The first includes a set of questioning prompts, i.e. a series of questions to promote reflective thinking for reflective writing or reflective journaling. The second is a series of guidelines and norms that can assist with reflective writing, feedback or critiquing.

A questioning prompt for reflecting on practice

- What do you think about this?
- What assumptions were you making at this point?
- Did you challenge the assumption of _____?
- Were you sceptical about the validity of this decision/conclusion?
- Which explanation is best supported by the intelligence?
- What other interventions could have been used?
- Was intuition involved in making this decision or coming to this conclusion?
- Did you reflect on the feasibility of _____?
- How did you arrive at this conclusion?
- How did you evaluate your thinking processes on _____?
- How did you evaluate your analysis of the data?
- How many other interventions/outcomes might have been considered in making your decision?
- What decisions would you make to manage this situation differently?
- What would the results look like?
- Did you trust your judgement?
- Did you consider other alternatives?
- What conclusions did you reach after examining your own critical, reflective thinking?

Source: Adapted from Van Aswegen.[114]

Guidelines and norms for reflective writing, feedback and critiquing

- A reflective journal is meant to support critical reflective learning and promote critical reflective practice.
- Reflections are neither right nor wrong, journals and reflective writings are about self-expression.
- Reflective writings/journals take on the voice and style of the practitioner – there is no correct writing style.
- Reflective writings often evoke more questions than answers. Questions help to focus on personal meaning and interpretation in the reflective moment.
- The question 'What are the implications of this reflection for my PHN practice?' can assist with professional development.
- Practitioners are encouraged to share and discuss chosen entries/writings with colleagues and others for feedback.
- Reflections are a personal experience. Critiques and mentoring relationships should provide a safe and supportive environment where the practitioner can share only what they feel safe about. Confidentiality should be maintained.
- Those who critique and mentor are not evaluators but rather guide, promote and challenge critical reflective thinking
- The response of those who critique/mentor should be non-judgemental and focused on supporting, motivating and guiding reflections and critical thinking.
- An arrangement about timing and respect between reflector and critique/mentor should be discussed and agreed to at the start of the relationship.
- Consider using the questioning prompt (tool 1) to promote and validate critical reflective thinking.

Source: Adapted from Harris.[113]

What is valorisation?

The term valorisation comes from from the French *valoriser* (to make useful, use or exploit)[115] and was adopted by the European Commission to describe the concept of 'building on achievements'. The European Commission define valorisation as:

> the process of disseminating and exploiting the results of projects with the view to optimising their impact, transferring them, integrating them in a sustainable way and using them actively in systems and practices at local, regional, national and European levels. (Directorate-General for Education and Culture. *Dissemination and exploitation of results*. ec.europa.eu/dgs/education_culture/valorisation/doc/def_en.pdf)

In reference to PHN intervention management valorisation is the transfer of the intelligence, learning and evaluation results gained from a PHN intervention to others, including the target population, key stakeholders, funding agencies and professional peers. Dissemination of intervention results may also involve local, regional or national media stories or advocacy to political and professional decision-makers. The process and extent of valorisation vary according to the intervention size, target population and strategies implemented.

Table 20.4   Key reasons for valorisation

Why have a valorisation plan?
• To improve/ensure sustainability of the intervention results.
• To enhance intervention organisation and management.
• To generate savings by not 'reinventing the wheel' and improve intervention planning.
• To indicate where further research and action is needed.
• To capitalise on and offer recognition of capacity and financial investments.
• To assist secure additional funding or managerial support for on-going activities.
• To influence decision-makers by using evaluation results as advocacy evidence.
• To assist with policy innovation and feed the policy process.
• To provide information for publicity.

Source: Adapted from Peberdy.[116]

Valorisation is an essential step in the PHN intervention management bi-cycle to ensure the active involvement of potential end-users and target groups during the intervention developments and to assist sustainability and progression of the intervention. Table 20.4 outlines the key reasons for developing the systematic dissemination and exploitation of results.

Targets of valorisation

Valorisation involves considering how best to communicate effectively and persuasively with a variety of groups and individuals. Valorisation largely seeks to influence people who are in a position to make decisions or take actions that will impact on the PHN issue, the intervention or similar interventions in other areas. Such people may include the target population, professional peers or politicians. The amount of time and effort spent, the strategies adopted and the groups and individuals to target will be largely political decisions according to the situation and context – knowing who makes what decisions is a crucial for successful valorisation. Table 20.5 outlines several groups who should be considered in valorisation.

Methods of valorisation

The most common method of sharing the evaluation results of a PHN intervention is through a project report. However, with many issues competing for people's attention an evaluation rarely is given a thorough reading. To be effective, the tools used in valorisation need to succeed in the challenging task of reaching and impacting on numerous, scattered audiences. Answering the questions 'Who needs to learn from the intervention experience?' and 'What do different groups and individuals needs to know about the evaluation results?' will influence the method employed for valorisation[116] using the information in Table 20.4 (about the different uses of intervention evaluation findings

Table 20.5 Different groups for consideration in valorisation

Potential valorisation audience	Example – breastfeeding intervention
Users and potential users, including both primary and secondary target groups	Participants – mothers and partners Maternal and child health nurses/ pharmacists
Key stakeholders involved in intervention delivery	Community workers Health workers Community members
Managers in key organisations	Community health manager(s) Manager of a non-for-profit community organisation Hospital executive
Professional bodies and peers	Nutrition organisations Breastfeeding/nursing mothers' association Nursing/midwifery organisations Informal/formal professional networks
Policy-makers and politicians	Local federal member Local government representatives Senior health/family services bureaucrats
Funding agencies	National/regional health board/department Health research institution Local philanthropic organisation
The media	Local newspaper Hospital/community health newsletter Local/regional radio

Source: Adapted from Peberdy.[116]

and learnings) and Table 20.3 (regarding who to target will clarify the range and nature of reaching the appropriate audiences).

Results from intervention evaluation can be qualitative or quantitative measures or a combination of the two. It is important to be highly selective with evaluation findings and to select consciously on the basis of the needs and interests of the audience.[116] For example, a fellow public health nutritionist as a specialist working in the field is likely to be interested in the details of how the intervention was implemented (process evaluation) and how the participants received and reacted to the intervention strategies (qualitative impact evaluation) as well as the impact on core nutrition-related behaviours, skills and knowledge. However, a journalist or policy-maker may only be interested in the intervention's impact and what action should be taken by decision-makers (quantitative impact/outcome evaluation and evaluation recommendations) as a result.

When thinking about who needs to know what, it is also important to respect time and areas of responsibility. How much od an individual's time and commitment/workload allocated to the PHN issue in question will help determine whether to provide a full report, a summary or arrange a meeting/presentation, and how best to focus the information provided about the intervention results. Completing a flow of information matrix can assist with developing a valorisation plan. Table 20.6 provides an example of a flow of information matrix for a nutrition intervention in secondary schools.

Table 20.6   Flow of information matrix

Who?	Role in intervention/ valorisation	What results?	How?
Teenagers and parents directly involved	Central in intervention planning and implementation	Full results and recommendations for future action	Meetings Newsletters Presentation
Teachers and school executive directly involved	Central in intervention planning and implementation	Full results and recommendations for future action	Meetings Newsletters Full or summary report Presentation
Nearby schools	Answer questions (control group)	Summary to create interest for potential action	Meetings Newsletters
Community workers	Coordinate and facilitate intervention planning, implementation and evaluation	Full results and recommendations for future action	Meetings Full project report
Local media	Can disseminate lessons learned	Summary of results	Media release Interviews
National-level education and health agencies and departments	Can disseminate lessons learned and support future action or policy change	Full results or summary	Meetings Presentations Summary report
Professional peers	Can support future action	Full results or summary	Conference presentations Professional networks Published papers

Source: Adapted from Peberdy.[116]

Presenting intervention results

Presenting the evaluation findings of a PHN intervention involves using the information and intelligence gathered to add colour and realism and conveying the impact and feelings of the intervention and the experience of the participants. Depending on the context and target group, written reports, newsletter articles, press releases, speeches, slide-shows and even drama can all be ways to communicate intervention results. Presentations that do not rely on the written word will be especially useful and appropriate with young children and populations whose literacy is low.[116]

Written reports

Valorisation always involves some form of written report. The written intervention or project report introduces the PHN problem and target population, explains the methodology adopted, presents the evaluation findings and whether the intervention goals and objectives were met, and finally provides conclusions and recommendations.

If the report is being submitted to a funding body, the format will usually be fixed. In other circumstances, or for a different audience, the length and structure of project report will be decided by the project team or project management committee. When determining the length and structure of a written project report it is wise to remember that the purpose of valorisation is to communicate the findings in a manner that attracts attention and gains credibility, not to switch off or drown the readers in a deluge of words.[11] It is also important to consider which aspects of evaluation (process, impact, outcome, capacity gains, economic assessment) are of most interest to the audience the report is targeted towards. Table 20.7 shows the general structure of a written intervention report.

Written reporting can also involve producing a press release, a newsletter article, a published paper or conference poster, or even a picture book or comic-strip (i.e. illustrations and words combined). As outlined above, the type of written reporting selected depends on the target audience and size of the intervention.

Oral reporting

An oral report can be a successful way of engaging an audience on the spot and conveying the findings of an intervention. Oral reporting commonly includes an account of some or all of the intervention objectives, the methodology and the main findings and recommendations. Visual aids (slides, participant quotes or photos) can be useful to help focus the audience on the key points. Visual aids should be clear, succinct and complement what is being said.[116]

Practice note

In some instances where an intervention has not been successful, project partners and funding agencies may be reluctant to undertake thorough valorisation fearing that the intervention may be considered a 'failure' and reflect negatively on the project partners and participants. However, it is important to valorise and share inconclusive or negative findings and learnings from these interventions to contribute to the broader body of PHN intelligence about what strategies do and do not work in given situations. Adding to the broader intelligence bank is vital for more effective and efficient PHN intervention delivery in the future.

Table 20.7   The general structure of a written report

Section	Description
Summary	Brief outline of the problem, target population, aim of the intervention, methodology of the intervention, key findings and recommendations. Maximum of one page.
Introduction	Describes the background and importance of the PHN problem, the target group(s) involved and the economic, political and strategic context of this particular intervention. May include the determinant analysis diagram and state the goals and objectives of the intervention.
Methodology	Outlines how the intervention was carried out, providing details of the strategies used and why these particular strategies were selected. Involves describing the intervention and evaluation design, sample, measurements and analysis methods employed.
Results	Present the quantitative and qualitative results, in detail and in summary form for clear comprehension. Use tables, graphs and diagrams to summarise the results.
Conclusions	Outline whether the goals and objectives of the intervention where met by providing a full interpretation of the intervention findings. Might involve answering the following questions: • What broad conclusion can be made from the intervention results? • Is the intervention of benefit? To whom? In what circumstances? • Which aspects of the intervention were most and least effective? • How do the results compare with other, similar interventions? • What are the key learnings about PHN interventions from this project? • What gaps in knowledge and understanding have been revealed? • What are the limitations of the intervention and/or evaluation and how do these limitations affect the conclusion?
Recommendations	Outlines what further action should be taken. Might involve answering the following questions: • What are the five main changes or additions that should be considered to improve the intervention? • Who would benefit most if the project were to be undertaken with another group? • What objectives might be changed or added to the project to expand its scope or effectiveness?

Source: Adapted from Peberdy.[116]

Key points

- Reflective practice is a constant process which involves thoughtful consideration of one's experiences to learn from and enhance practice. By spending time exploring why they acted as they did, what occurred in the group and what the participants' and stakeholders' response was, the practitioner can learn and improve future activity and practice.
- Reflective practice becomes a source of intelligence which is as useful as objective intelligence and feeds into the continuation of the PHN intervention management bi-cycle into the next intelligence stage.
- Reflective practice is a companion or precursor to professional development by assessing the congruency of practice behaviour with personal/professional values and beliefs, and assisting autonomous practice through self-monitoring and accountability. Methods of reflective practice include reflective writing and journaling, critique and mentoring.
- Valorisation is the transfer of the intelligence, learnings and evaluation results gained from a PHN intervention to others, including the target population, key stakeholders, funding agencies and professional peers.
- Valorisation is an essential step in the PHN intervention management bi-cycle to ensure the active involvement of potential end-users and target groups during the intervention developments and to assist sustainability and progression of the intervention.

Appendices

Appendix 1

Intervention plan template

Intervention summary statement

Provide a summary description of the intervention planned.
A reader should be able to read and answer questions about the intervention:

- *Why?*
- *What?*
- *How?*
- *Who?*
- *By when?*

Approximately 300 words

Community analysis

Provide a summary description of the community this intervention plan relates to. Include a description of community attributes

Approximately 300 words

Problem analysis

Provide a summary description of the problem this intervention plan relates to. Include a description of:

- *The nature, severity and scale of problem.*
- *The distribution of problem?*

Approximately 500 words

Practical Public Health Nutrition, first edition. Roger Hughes and Barrie M. Margetts. Published 2011 by Blackwell Publishing Ltd. © 2011 Roger Hughes and Barrie M. Margetts.

Stakeholder analysis

Provide a summary description of the major stakeholders related to the problem being addressed:

- What we know about the target group, description, etc.
- Motivation and opportunities of the target group
- Accessibility and engagement with the target group

Approximately 300 words

Determinant analysis

Provide a summary description of the determinant analysis you have conducted demonstrating an understanding of the problem:

- *What are the determinants of the problem?*
- *What determinants are amenable to change?*
- *How have determinants been prioritised or selected for change?*
- *What theoretical models or assumptions are being used?*

Insert determinant analysis diagram and describe analysis of the causative relationship between determinants and problem.

Approximately 400 words

Mandates for action

Provide a summary of existing mandates for action that support investment in your intervention.

Approximately 300 words

Existing capacity for action

Provide a summary of existing capacity and capacity gaps that support your call for extra resources and investment to support problem solving.

Approximately 300 words

Project partners and governance

Provide a summary of who and how you plan to establish intervention governance structures that include key stakeholders and assist decision making.

Use diagrams as required.

Approximately 300 words

Goal and objectives

Insert action statements

- *Goal statement.*
- *Are objectives SMART?*
- *Do objectives fit the analysis?*
- *Are the objectives are acceptable?*
- *Are the objectives feasible?*

Intervention research

Summarise the intelligence from previous interventions (intervention research) that demonstrates you have considered the learnings from previous effort. How has this informed your strategy mix?

Limit to 250 words

Strategy mix

Summarise the rationale and describe the strategy mix

- *Describe strategy mix*
- *Do strategies fit with objectives (what is the logic model)?*
- *Why do we think they have merit and are likely to work?*
- *Are strategies supported by intervention research evidence?*

Evaluation plan

Describe the evaluation plan, specifically describing methods, howthe evaluation relates to goals and objectives and the types of evaluation:

- *Process.*
- *Impact.*
- *Outcome.*
- *Capacity.*
- *Economic evaluation.*

What are the evaluation research questions?

What theoretical frameworks are used?

How are we accounting for confounding effects on evaluation results? (intervention vs. control comparisons, etc.)

Evaluation stage	Method	Description of data collection/ analysis method	Data type	Answers Question No?	Output/ Dissemination
Formative					
Process					
Impact					
Outcome					
Capacity					
Economic					

Activity planning

Work package descriptions

Activity/Task	Method	Who	When

Budget

Project costs

Item	Costs[1]
1. Investment by permanent staff (FTE estimates only)	
2. Project budget:	
a) Temporary project staff (insert level, FTE and time period)	
b) Associated non-labour and corporate overheads	
c) Other (itemise)	
Project budget – total	

Resource contribution from stakeholders

Estimated margin of error

Cost implications post-project

Justification

---

[1] If project is multi-year, add additional columns and provide costs for each financial year.

Project schedule – timelines

Strategy/ Activity	Accountable Officer/s	Duration	Months (adjust timeframe as necessary)											
			Jan	Feb	Mar	Apr	May	June	July	Aug	Sept	Oct	Nov	Dec
Project strategy implementation / finalisation activities														
Project management activities														

Risk management

What do you foresee might go wrong, and how will you plan to manage?

Risk	Risk Management Activities	
	Preventive	Contingent

Communication management (valorisation)

What plan do you have to keep stakeholders informed and to ensure project effects/ impacts are shared and utilised?

What?	How?	With/To Whom?	When/How often?

References/intelligence sources

Insert references to intelligence used in this document

Appendix 2

Capacity building analysis tool

Use this checklist to analyse capacity before, during and after an intervention and to help focus capacity building effort.

LEADERSHIP	Contribution to capacity					Evidence
	1 Nil obvious	2 Limited	3 Average	4 Significant	5 Very significant	
Political	Issue /project has no obvious political support	Politicians aware of project but have limited involvement	General political awareness and limited support	Politicians at one level championing the project/issue	Politicians at numerous levels championing the project/issue	
Organisational	No issue-specific leadership within local organisations	Local organisations aware of issues with limited actions to address it	Average issue-specific leadership in one local organisation and others aware of issues but only acting in a limited manner to address it	Numerous local organisations leading action and driving change	Multiple organisations at different levels working collaboratively to lead action on issue and drive change	
Community	No issue-specific leadership obvious within community	Limited number of community members aware of issues and acting in limited manner to address it	Average issue-specific leadership by a few community members and others aware of issues but only acting in a limited manner to address it	Numerous members of the community leading action and driving change	Many members across different levels of community leading action and driving change	
Workforce	No issue specific leadership obvious within workforce	Limited number of practitioners in the workforce aware of issues and acting in a limited manner to address it	Average issue-specific leadership by workforce practitioners and others aware of issues but only acting in a limited manner to address it	Numerous practitioners in a limited number of workforce disciplines leading action and driving change	Workforce practitioners from multiple service disciplines leading action and driving change	
Project	One-sided or vested interests in project leadership, undemocratically chosen and unrelated to common interests	Community organisation represents the community, but health staff work independently of this organisation	Community organisation functioning in collaboration with health staff, but without wide support from the community	Active community organisation but acknowledges lack of input from marginalised sections of community. Tends to lack heterogeneity in leadership	Community organisation fully represents variety of interests in community and is motivated out of concern for health of all of its population in the future.	

RESOURCES	Contribution to capacity					Evidence
	1 Nil obvious	2 Limited	3 Average	4 Significant	5 Very significant	
RESOURCE MOBILISATION — Community	External funding only, community raises/contributes no obvious resources	External funding and small amount of resources raised/contributed by community	External funding and fair amount of resources raised/contributed by community	External funding and significant amount of resources raised/contributed by community	External funding and extensive amount of resources raised/contributed by community	
Services & Programmes	General services but no obvious investment in issue specific services and programmes	Limited investment in issue specific services and programs	Average investment in issue-specific services and programmes	Significant investment in issue-specific services and programmes	Extensive investment in issue-specific services and programmes	
RESOURCE ALLOCATION — Human resources	No obvious investment in health staff specific to the issue	Limited investment in generic health staff and specialists specific to the issue	Average investment in generic health staff, and specialists specific to the issue	Significant investment in generic health staff and specialists specific to the issue	Very significant investment in generic health staff and specialists specific to the issue	
Research	No obvious investment in generic health research and dissemination	Limited investment in generic health research and dissemination	Average investment in generic and issue-specific health research and dissemination	Significant investment in generic health research and dissemination, and limited investment in issue-specific research and dissemination	Extensive investments in generic and issue-specific health research and dissemination	
Infrastructure	No obvious investment in physical infrastructure to support generic health promotion	Limited investment in physical infrastructure to support generic health promotion	Average investment in physical infrastructure to support generic and issue-specific health promotion	Significant investment in infrastructure to support generic health promotion, and limited investment in infrastructure to support issue specific health promotion	Extensive investment in infrastructure to support generic and issue specific health promotion across multiple sectors	

PARTNERSHIPS	Contribution to capacity					Evidence
	1 Nil obvious	2 Limited	3 Average	4 Significant	5 Very significant	
Networks	There are no obvious existing networks that relate to the issue	There are limited existing networks that relate to the issue	There are average existing networks that relate to the issue	There are significant existing networks that relate to the issue	There are very significant existing networks that relate to the issue	
Membership	There is no obvious collaboration or partnerships formed to support the issue	The partnership includes only a limited membership at one level with a small focus on the issue	The partnership includes an average membership with some focus on the issue	The partnership includes a significant membership across a number of levels with significant focus on the issue	There is extensive collaboration between partners across many levels with major support for issue	
Shared vision	There is wide disagreement within the partnership as to their purpose and mission	Only a limited number of members of the partnership share the same vision	Many members of the partnership share the same vision as each other, but not that of the external community	A significant proportion of the partnership share the same vision as each other and that of the external community	All members of the partnership share the same vision as each other and the external community to support the issue	
Resource exchange	There is no obvious exchange of resources between partners	There is limited exchange of resources between partners	There is a fair exchange of resources between partners at the same level	There is significant exchange of resources between partners but rarely across levels	There is extensive exchange of resources between partners across all levels	
Communication	There are no obvious lines of communication between partners	There are limited lines of communication between partners, and they rarely relate to the issue	There is fair communication between partners at the same level on a limited range of topics relating to the issue	There is significant communication between partners across levels on a significant range of topics relating to the issue	There is extensive collaboration between partners across all levels and all topics relating to the issue	

COMMUNITY ENGAGEMENT	Contribution to capacity					Evidence
	1 Nil obvious	2 Limited	3 Average	4 Significant	5 Very significant	
Problem identification	There is no obvious identification of the problem by the community	There is limited identification of the issue/problem by the community	There is some identification of the issue by a few sections of the community	There is significant identification of the issue by most sections of the community	There is extensive identification of the issue by a broad representation of the community	
Strategy identification	The community does not obviously identify strategies to deal with the issue	Small sections of the community identify limited strategies to deal with the issue	Some sections of the community identify average strategies to deal with the issue	Many sections of the community identify a significant range of strategies to deal with the issue	A major proportion of the community identify extensive strategies to deal with the issue	
Planning involvement	The community has no obvious involvement in planning interventions to deal with the issue	Small sections of the community have limited involvement in planning interventions to ceal with the issue	Some sections of the community have average involvement in planning interventions to deal with the issue	Many sections of the community have significant involvement in planning interventions to deal with the issue	A major proportion of the community has very significant involvement in planning interventions to deal with the issue	
Implementation	The community has no obvious involvement in the implementation of strategies to deal with the issue	Small sections of te community have limited involvement in the implementation of strategies to deal with the issue	Some sections of the community have average involvement in the implementation of strategies to deal with the issue	Many sections of the community have significant involvement in the implementation of strategies to deal with the issue	A major proportion of the community has extensive involvement in the implementation of strategies to deal with the issue	
Service use	The community does not obviously participate in programmes relevant to the issue	Small sections of the community participate in a lmited number of programmes relevant to the issue	Some sections of the community participate in an average number of programmrs relevant to the issue	Many sections of the community participate in a significant number of programmes relevant to the issue	A major proportion of the community participate extensively in programmes relevant to the issue	

WORKFORCE DEVELOPMENT	Contribution to capacity					Evidence
	1 Nil obvious	2 Limited	3 Average	4 Significant	5 Very significant	
Size and composition	There is a very small workforce with no practitioners obviously trained/experienced in the issue	There is a small workforce with a limited number of practitioners trained/experienced in the issue	There is a fair-sized workforce with an average number of practitioners trained/experienced in the issue	There is a large workforce with a significant number of practitioners trained/experienced in the issue	There is a very large workforce with an extensive number of practitioners trained/experienced in the issue	
Competencies/ Preparedness	The workforce has no obvious knowledge, skills or abilities to deal with the issue	The workforce has limited knowledge, skills and abilities to deal with the issue	The workforce has fair knowledge, skills and abilities to deal with the issue	The workforce has significant knowledge, skills and abilities to deal with the issue	The workforce has very significant knowledge, skills and abilities to deal with the issue	
Practices	Workforce actions are not obviously based on intelligence or practice	Workforce practices are limited, with little emphasis on intelligence or CPD opportunities	There are average workforce practices, with an fair emphasis on intelligence and CPD opportunities	There are significant workforce practices, with a large emphasis on intelligence and CPD opportunities	There are very significant workforce practices, with a major emphasis on intelligence and CPD opportunities	
Management/ Organisation	The organisational structure and management of the workplace does not obviously support best practice	The organisational structure and management of the workplace has limited support for best practice	The organisational structure and management of the workplace has average support for best practice	The organisational structure and management of the workplace has significant support for best practice	The organisational structure and management of the workplace has very significant support for best practice	
Community engagement in practice	There is no obvious consultation between any levels of workforce and the community in order to improve practice	There is limited consultation between workforce and community in order to improve practice	There is average consultation between some levels of workforce and community in order to improve practice	There is significant consultation between most levels of workforce and community in order to improve practice	There is very significant consultation between all levels of workforce and community in order to improve practice	

ORGANISATIONAL DEVELOPMENT	Contribution to capacity					Evidence
	1 Nil obvious	2 Limited	3 Average	4 Significant	5 Very significant	
Mandates (policy)	There are no obvious organisational policies that support action on the issue/problem	There are limited organisational policies that support action on the issue/problem	There are average organisational policies that support action on the issue/problem	There are significant organisational policies that support action on the issue/problem	There are very significant organisational policies that support action on the issue/problem	
Plans	There is no obvious organisational planning to address the issue	There is limited organisational planning to address the issue	There is average organisational planning to address the issue	There is significant organisational planning to address the issue	There is very significant organisational planning to address the issue	
Organisational structure	The organisational structures do not obviously support workers to fulfil their roles	The organisational structures provide limited support for workers to fulfil their roles	The organisational structures provide average support for workers to fulfil their roles	The organisational structures provide significant support for workers to fulfil their roles	The organisational structures provide very significant support for workers to fulfil their roles	
Learning culture	The organisation does not have an obvious learning culture for research, CPD, and best practice	The organisation has a small learning culture or limited quality	The organisation has a average learning culture of fair quality	The organisation has a large learning culture of significant quality	The organisation has an extensive learning culture of very significant quality	
Coordination/ Linkages	The organisation has no obvious links or coordination with partners at any level	There is limited coordination between the organisation and other collaborators	There is average coordination between the organisation and collaborators from a few levels	There is significant coordination between the organisation and collaborators from many levels	There is extensive coordination between the organisation and collaborators from all levels	
Responsiveness	The organisation has no obvious ability to mobilise action to address the specific issue/problem	The organisation has limited ability to mobilise action to address the specific issue/problem	The organisation has an average ability to mobilise action to address the specific issue/problem	The organisation has significant ability to mobilise action to address the specific issue/problem	The organisation has extensive ability to mobilise action to address the specific issue/problem	

INTELLIGENCE	Contribution to capacity					Evidence
	1 Nil obvious	2 Limited	3 Average	4 Significant	5 Very significant	
Needs assessment	There was no obvious input into the needs assessment phase of the project/issue	There was limited input into the needs assessment phase of the project/issue	There was average input into the needs assessment phase of the project/issue	There was significant input into the needs assessment phase of the project/issue	There was extensive input into the needs assessment phase of the project/issue	
Monitoring and surveillance systems	There are no obvious surveillance systems in place to monitor general public health programs or those specific to the issue	There are limited surveillance systems in place to monitor general public health programmes and those specific to the issue	There are average surveillance systems in place to monitor general public health programmes and those specific to the issue	There are significant surveillance systems in place to monitor general public health programmes and those specific to the issue	There are extensive surveillance systems in place to monitor general public health programmes and those specific to the issue	
Intelligence-based strategies	Strategies are not based on any obvious intelligence or evidence	Strategies are based on limited intelligence and evidence	Strategies are based on average intelligence and evidence	Strategies are based on significant intelligence and evidence	Strategies are based on very significant intelligence and evidence	
Knowledge transfer	The is no obvious evidence of intelligence transfer between practitioners, the community and academics	There is limited evidence of intelligence transfer between practitioners, the community and academics	There is average evidence of intelligence transfer between practitioners, the community and academics	There is significant evidence of intelligence transfer between practitioners, the community and academics	There is very significant evidence of intelligence transfer between practitioners, the community and academics	

PROJECT MANAGEMENT	Contribution to capacity					Evidence
	1 Nil obvious	2 Limited	3 Average	4 Significant	5 Very significant	
Problem analysis	There is no obvious evidence of the project managements investment in problem analysis and identification	There is limited evidence of the project managements investment in problem analysis and identification	There is average evidence of the project managements investment in problem analysis and identification	There is significant evidence of the project managements investment in problem analysis and identification	There is very significant evidence of the project management investment in problem analysis and identification	
Stakeholder engagement	Decisions regarding project management are made by individuals only	Decisions regarding project management are made by a small number of stakeholders	Decisions regarding project management are made by an average representation of stakeholders	Decisions regarding project management are made by a large number of stakeholders	Decisions regarding project management are made by an extensive number of stakeholders	
Determinant analysis	There is no obvious evidence of the project managements investment in determinant analysis	There is limited evidence of the project managements investment in determinant analysis	There is average evidence of the project managements investment in determinant analysis	There is significant evidence of the project managements investment in determinant analysis	There is very significant evidence of the project management investment in determinant analysis	
Target group identification	There is no obvious evidence of the project managements investment in target group identification	There is limited evidence of the project managements investment in target group identification	There is average evidence of the project managements investment in target group identification	There is significant evidence of the project managements investment in target group identification	There is very significant evidence of the project management investment in target group identification	

Continued

PROJECT MANAGEMENT	Contribution to capacity					Evidence
	1 Nil obvious	2 Limited	3 Average	4 Significant	5 Very significant	
Objectives	There is no obvious evidence that objectives are based on SMART objective design	There is limited evidence that objectives are based on SMART objective design	There is average evidence that objectives are based on SMART objective design	There is significant evidence that objectives are based on SMART objective design	There is very significant evidence that objectives are based on SMART objective design	
Strategy mix	There is no obvious evidence that project management based interventions on a mix of strategies	There is limited evidence that project management based interventions on a mix of strategies	There is average evidence that project management based interventions of a mix of strategies	There is significant evidence that project management based interventions of a mix of strategies	There is very significant evidence that project management based interventions of a mix of strategies	
Implementation	There are no obvious implementation plan in place	There are limited implementation plans in place	There are average implementation plans in place	There are significant implementation plans in place	There are very significant implementation plans in place	
Evaluation	There are no obvious methods in place for evaluation of strategies	There are limited methods in place for evaluation of strategies	There are average methods in place for evaluation of strategies	There are significant methods in place for both process and effect evaluation of strategies	There are very significant methods in place for both process and effect evaluation of strategies	
Sustainability	There is no obvious evidence of project managements consideration of sustainability of the programme once funding ceases	There is limited evidence of project managements consideration of sustainability of the programme once funding ceases	There is average evidence of project managements consideration of sustainability of the programme once funding ceases	There is significant evidence of project managements consideration of sustainability of the programme once funding ceases	There is very significant evidence of project managements consideration of sustainability of the programme once funding ceases	

References

1. FAO/WFP, *The state of food insecurity in the world. Economic crisies – impacts and lessons learned*, FAO, Editor. 2009, FAO: Rome.
2. Victora, C. et al., Maternal and child under-nutrition: consequences for adult health and human capital. *Lancet*, 2008, **371**: pp. 340–357.
3. Black, R. et al., Maternal and child under-nutrition: global and regional exposures and health consequences. *Lancet*, 2008, **371**: pp. 243–260.
4. Bhutta, Z. et al., Maternal and child under-nutrition: what works? Interventions for maternal and child under-nutrition and survival. *Lancet*, 2008, **371**: pp. 417–440.
5. Morris, S., Cogill, B. & Uauy, R., Effective international action against under-nutrition: why has it proven so diffi cult and what can be done to accelerate progress? *Lancet*, 2008, **371**: pp. 608–621.
6. Bryce, J. et al., Maternal and child under-nutrition: effective action at national level. *Lancet*, 2008, **371**: pp. 510–526.
7. WHO, *Diet, nutrition and the prevention of chronic diseases. Report of a joint WHO/FAO expert consultation.* WHO Technical Report Series **916**.
8. Hughes, R. & Somerset, S., Definitions and conceptual frameworks for public health and community nutrition: a discussion paper. *Aust J Nutr Diet*, 1997, **54**(1): pp. 40–45.
9. Rogers, B. & Schlossman, N., 'Public nutrition': the need for cross-disciplinary breadth in the education of applied nutrition professionals. *Food and Nutrition Bulletin*, 1997, **18**(2): pp. 120–133.
10. Landman, J., Buttriss, J. & Margetts, B., Curriculum design for professional development in public health nutrition in Britain. *Public Health Nutrition*, 1998, **1**(1): pp. 69–74.
11. Yngve, A. et al., Effective promotion of healthy nutrition and physical activity in Europe requires skilled and competent people; European Master's Programme in Public Health Nutrition. *Public Health Nutrition*, 1999, **2**(3a): pp. 449–452.
12. Johnson, D. et al., Public health nutrition practice in the United States. *J Am Diet Assoc*, 2001, **101**(5): pp. 529–534.

13. Beaudry, M. & Delisle, H., Public('s) nutrition. *Public Health Nutrition*, 2005. **8**: pp. 743–748.

14. Hughes, R., Definitions for public health nutrition: A developing consensus. *Public Health Nutrition*, 2003, **6**(6): pp. 615–620.

15. Cannon, G. & Leitzmann, C., The new nutrition science project. *Public Health Nutrition*, 2005, **8**: pp. 673–694.

16. World Health Organisation, Ottawa charter for health promotion. *Health Promotion*, 1986, **4**: pp. ii–v.

17. NPHP, *Public health practice in Australia today – core functions*, 2001. Melbourne: National Public Health Partnership.

18. USDHHS, *The essential public health services work group of the Core Public Health Functions Steering Committee*, 1995. Office of the Assistant Secretary of Health.

19. Hughes, R., A socio-ecological analysis of the determinants of national public health nutrition workforce capacity: Australia as a case study. *Family & Community Health*, 2006, **29**: pp. 55–67.

20. Hughes, R., Public health nutrition workforce development: an intelligence based blueprint for Australia, in *School of Health Science*, 2003, Gold Coast: Griffith University.

21. Hughes, R., Practices overview, in M. Lawrence & A. Worsley, eds., *Public health nutrition: from principles to practice*, 2007. Crows Nest: Allen & Unwin, pp. 265–272.

22. Ocklers, L., Gibbs, T. & Duncan, M., Developing health science students into integrated health professionals: a practical tool for learning. *BMC Medical Education*, 2007, **7**: p. 45.

23. Margetts, B., An overview of public health nutrition, in B. M. M. Gibney, B. M. Margetts, M. J. Kearney & L. Arab, eds.. *Public Health Nutrition*, 2004, Oxford: Blackwell: pp. 1–25.

24. Jonsson, U., A conceptual approach to understanding and explanation of hunger and malnutrition in society, in *Hunger and Society*, 1988, New York: Cornell International Monograph Series.

25. Baillie, E. et al., A capacity-building conceptual framework for public health nutrition practice. *Public Health Nutr*, 2009, **12**(8): pp. 1031–1038.

26. Hawe, P. et al., Working invisibly: health workers talk about capacity-building in health promotion. *Health Promotion International*, 1998, **13**(4): pp. 285–295.

27. Green, L. & Raeburn, J., Community wide change: theory and practice, in N. Bracht, ed., *Health promotion at the community level*, 1990. Palo Alto, CA: Sage.

28. Robinson, K. & Elliott, S., The practice of community development approaches in heart health promotion. *Health Education Research*, 2000, **15**: pp. 219–231.

29. Naidoo, J. & Willis, J., *Health promotion – foundations for practice*, 2nd edition. 2000. London: Harcourt.

30. Kelly, K. & Van Vlaenderen, H., Dynamics of participation in a community health project. *Social Science and Medicine*, 1996, **42**: pp. 1235–1246.

31. Dalziel, Y., Community development as a public health function. in S. Cowley, ed., *Public health in policy and practice: a source book for health visitors and community nurses*, 2002. Edinburgh: Baillière Tindall, pp. 217–238.

32. Rifkin, S., A framework linking community empowerment and health equity: it is a matter of choice. *Journal of Health Population Nutrition*, 2003, **21**: pp. 168–180.

33. Hancock, T., People, partnerships and human progress: building community capital. *Health Promotion International*, 2001, **16**: pp. 275–280.

34. Armstrong, D., A survey of community gardens in upstate New York: implications for health promotion and community development. *Health Place*, 2000, **6**: pp. 319–327.

35. Laverack, G. & Labonte, R., A planning framework for community empowerment goals within health promotion. *Health Policy Plan*, 2000. **15**(3): pp. 255–262.

36. Francis K. et al., *Community as partner: theory and practice in nursing*, 2007. Sydney: Lippincott Williams & Wilkins.

37. Talbot, L. & Verrinder, G., *Promoting health: the primary health care approach*, 3rd edition. 2005. Marrickville: Elsevier Churchill Livingstone.

38. Bradshaw, J., The concept of social need. *New Society*, March 1972: pp. 641–643.

39. Ryan, D., Mannix-McNamara, P. & Deasy, C., *Health promotion in Ireland – principles, practice and research*, 2006. Dublin: Gill & Macmillan.

40. UNCF (2008) *SWOT analysis*.

41. Brugha, R. & Varvasovskyz, Z., Stakeholder analysis: a review. *Health Policy and Planning*, 2000, **15**: pp. 239–345.

42. Varvasovskyz, Z. & Brugha, R., How to do (or not to do) … a stakeholder analysis. *Health Policy and Planning*, 2000, **15**: pp. 338-345.

43. GTZ, *Capacity Building Needs Assessment (CBNA) in the Regions (version 2.0) Module B. Methods and instruments for the capacity building cycle*. 2005, Jakarta: Deutsche Gesellschaft für Technische Zusammenarbeit (GTZ).

44. Lobstein, T., Can we prevent childhood obesity? *SCN Newsletter*, 2008, **29**.

45. NPHP, *A planning framework for public health practice – a system perspective*, 1999. Canberra: Commonwealth Department of Health and Aged Care.

46. Green, L. & Kreuter, M., eds., *Health promotion planning: an educational and environmental approach*, 1991. Mayfield: Mountain View.

47. Miilunpalo, S., Evidence and theory based health promotion of health-enhancing physical activity. *Public Health Nutrition*, 2001, **4**: pp. 725–728.

48. Miller, M. & Stafford, H., *Framework trial to develop an intervention portfolio to promote fruit and vegetables – summary report to the National Public Health Partnership* 2000. Canberra.

49. Zenk, S. N. et al., Fruit and vegetable intake in African Americans: income and store characteristics. *Am J Prev Med*, 2005, **29**(1): pp. 1–9.

50. Goodman, R. et al., Identifying and defining the dimensions of community capacity to provide a basis for measurement. *Health Education and Behavior*, 1998, **25**(3): pp. 258–278.

51. Horton, D. et al., Evaluating capacity development: experiences from research and development organisations around the world, in *The Netherlands: International Service for National Agriculture Research/International Development Research Centre*, 2003.

52. Baillie, E. et al., A capacity building conceptual framework for public health nutrition practice. *Public Health Nutrition*, 2009, **12**(8): pp. 1031–1038.

53. NSW Health, *A Framework for Building Capacity to Improve Health*, 2001. Sydney: NSW Health Department.

54. Ebbesen, L. S. et al., Issues in measuring health promotion capacity in Canada: a multi-province perspective. *Health Promot Int*, 2004, **19**(1): pp. 85–94.

55. Naidoo, J. & Wills, J., eds., *Public health and health promotion*. 2nd edition, 2005. London: Baillière Tindall.

56. Tones, K. & Green, J., Healthy public policy, in *Health promotion – planning and strategies*, 2004. London. Sage: pp. 175–207.

57. Walt, G., ed., *Health policy: An introduction to process and power*, 1994. London: Zed Books.

58. FAO/WHO, *World Declaration on Nutrition*. 1992, Rome: FAO/WHO.

59. WHO, *The First Action Plan for Food and Nutrition Policy, WHO European Region, 2000–2005*, 2000, Copenhagen: World Health Organisation Regional Office for Europe.

60. WHO, *Global Strategy on Diet, Physical Activity and Health, Resolution of the Fifty-seventh World Health Assembly. WHA 57.17*. 2004, Geneva: World Health Organisation.

61. WHO, *Comparative analysis of nutrition policies in the WHO European Region*, 2006, Copenhagen: World Health Organisation Regional Office for Europe.

62. World Health Organisation, The Jakarta Declaration on leading health promotion into the 21st century. *Health Prom Int*, 1997, **12**: pp. 261–264.

63. Tones, K. & Green, J., Healthy public policy, in *Health promotion – planning and strategies*, 2004. London: Sage: pp. 175–207.

64. WHO, *Bangkok Charter for health promotion in a globalised world. Sixth Global Conference on Health Promotion*, 2005. Bangkok: World Health Organisation.

65. French, S., Population approaches to promote healthful eating behaviours, in D. Crawford and R. Jeffrey, ed., *Obesity prevention and public health*, 2005. London: Oxford University Press: p. 103.

66. Keller, L. et al., Assessment, program planning, and evaluation in population-based public health practice. *J Public Health Management Practice*, 2002, **8**(5): pp. 30–43.

67. Tilford, S., Evidence-based health promotion. *Health Education Research*, 2000, **15**: pp. 659–663.

68. NPHP, *A planning framework for public health practice – a system perspective*, 1999. Canberra: Australian Commonwealth Department of Health and Aged Care.

69. Pickett, G. & Hanlon, J., eds., *Public heath: administration and practice*, 1990. Missouri: Times Mirror/Mosby College Publishing.

70. Swinburn, B., Egger, G. & Raza, F., Dissecting obesogenic environments: the development and application of a framework for identifying and prioritising environmental interventions for obesity. *Preventive Medicine*, 1999, **29**: pp. 563–570.

71. DHS, *ACE-Obesity: assessing cost effectiveness of obesity interventions in children and adolescents – summary results*, 2006. Melbourne: Victorian Government Department of Human Services.

72. Prevention, C.C.f.O., *A comprehensive approach to obesity prevention using the ANGELO framework. 2002*, 2002. Melbourne: World Health Organisation Collaborating Centre for Obesity Prevention.

73. Stanley, S. & Stein, D., Health Watch 2000: community health assessment in South Central Ohio. *Journal of Community Health Nursing*, 1998, **15**: pp. 225–236.

74. Hughes, R., Baillie, E. & Nalatu, S., Stakeholder engagement in intervention design in a community-based nutrition and physical activity promotion intervention targeting disadvantaged mothers in Australia, in *Proceedings Dietitians of Canada National Conference*, 2007. Vancouver.

75. Haby, M. et al., A new approach to assessing the health benefit from obesity interventions in children and adolescents: the assessing cost-effectiveness in obesity project. *International Journal of Obesity*, 2006, **30**: pp. 1463–1475.

76. Naidoo, J. & Willis, J., eds., *Health promotion – foundations for practice*, 2nd edition, 2000. London: Harcourt.

77. Oshaug, A., *Planning and managing community nutrition work: manual for personnel involved in community nutrition. 1992*, 1992. Copenhagen: World Health Organisation Regional Office for Europe.

78. WHO/FAO/EI, *WHO information series on school health – Document 4: Healthy nutrition: an essential element of a health-promoting school*, 1998, Geneva: World Health Organisation.

79. THCU, *Introduction to health promotion program planning*, 2001. Toronto: Centre for Health Promotion, University of Toronto.

80. Tones, K. & Tilford, S. eds., *Health promotion: effectiveness, efficiency and equity*. 2001, London: Chapman & Hall.

81. Hyman, H. ed., *Health planning: a systematic approach*, 1982. Rockville, MD: Aspen Systems.

82. Rossi, P., Freeman, H. & Lipsey, M., eds., *Evaluation: a systematic approach*, 1999. Thousand Oaks, CA: Sage.

83. Smith, M., ed., *Evaluability assessment: a practical approach*, 1989. Norwell: Kluwer Academic.

84. Taylor-Powell, E. & Henert, E., *Developing a logic model: teaching and training guide*, 2008. Madison, WI: University of Wisconsin-Extension.

85. THCU, *Logic models: workbook*, 2001. Toronto: The Health Communication Unit, University of Toronto.

86. Macaskill, L. et al., An evaluability assessment to develop a restaurant health promotion program in Canada. *Health Promotion International*, 2000, **15**: pp. 57–69.

87. TasGov, Project Business Plan (small) – Template and Guide, version 2.1, in D.o.P.a. Cabinet, ed., *Tasmanian Government Project Management Framework*, 2005. Hobart: Department of Premier and Cabinet.

88. WHO, *Health programme evaluation: guiding principles*. 1981, Geneva: World Health Organisation.

89. Hawe, P., Degeling, D. & Hall, J., eds., *Evaluating health promotion: a health worker's guide*, 1990. Sydney: MacLennan and Petty.

90. Thurston, W. & Potvin, L., Evaluability assessment: a tool for incorporating evaluation in social change programmes. *Evaluation*, 2003, **9**: pp. 453–469.

91. Ryan, D., Mannix McNamara, P. & Deasy, C., eds., Evaluation, in *Health promotion in Ireland: principles, practice and research*, 2006. Dublin: Gill & Macmillan.

92. Kunreuther, H., Risk analysis and risk management in an uncertain world. *Risk Analysis*, 2002, **22**: pp. 655–664.

93. Rosenmoller, M., Sachon, M. & Ribera, J., Risk management perception and communication in health care, in M. Davies & W. Macdowall, eds., *Health Promotion Theory*, 2006. Buckingham: Open University Press.

94. McLeod, J., *The partnerships analysis tool: for partners in health promotion*, 2003. Melbourne: Victorian Health Promotion Foundation.

95. Nutbeam, D. & Bauman, A., eds., *Evaluation in a nutshell: a practical guide to the evaluation of health promotion programmes*, 2006. Sydney: McGraw-Hill.

96. Platt, S. et al., Applying process evaluation, in M. Thorogood & Y. Coombes, eds., *Evaluating health promotion: practice and methods*, 2nd edition, 2004. New York: Oxford University Press.

97. Saunders, R., Evans, M. & Joshi, P., Developing a process-evaluation plan for assessing health promotion program implementation: a how-to guide. *Health Promotion Practice*, 2005, **6**: pp. 134–147.

98. Thorogood, M. & Coombes, Y., *Evaluating health promotion: practice and methods*, 2004. New York: Oxford University Press.

99. Gibbon, M., Labonte, R. & Laverack, G., Evaluating community capacity. *Health and Social Care in the Community*, 2002, **10**(6): pp. 485–491.

100. Bjaras, G., Haglund, B. & Rifkin, S., A new approach to community participation assessment. *Health Promotion International*, 1991, **6**(3): pp. 199–206.

101. Richardson, J., Economic evaluation of health promotion: friend or foe. *Australian and New Zealand Journal of Public Health*, 1998, **22**: pp. 247–253.

102. Ganz, M., The economic evaluation of obesity interventions: its time has come. *Obesity Research*, 2003, **11**: pp. 1275–1277.

103. Godfrey, C., Economic evaluation if health promotion, in I. Rootman et al., eds., *Evaluation in health promotion: principles and perspectives*, 2001. Copenhagen: World Health Organisation Regional Publications European Series.

104. Tones, K. & Tilford, S., *Health promotion: effectiveness, efficiency and equity*, 3rd edition 2001. Cheltenham: Nelson Thornes.

105. Stevens, W., Economic evaluation of health promotion interventions, in M. Thorogood & Y. Coombes, eds., *Evaluating health promotion: practice and methods*, 2004. New York: Oxford University Press.

106. Robroek, S., Bredt, F. & Burodf, A., The (cost-) effectiveness of an individually tailored long-term worksite health promotion programme on physical activity and nutrition: design of a pragmatic cluster randomised control trial. *BioMed Central Public Health*, 2007, **7**: pp. 259–270.

107. Gusi, N. et al., Cost-utility of a walking programme for moderately depressed, obese or overweight elderly women in primary care: a randomised controlled trial. *BioMed Central Public Health*, 2007, **8**: pp. 231–241.

108. Wang, L. et al., Economic evaluation of a school-based obesity prevention program. *Obesity Research*, 2003, **11**: pp. 1313–1324.

109. Schön, D. ed., *The reflective practitioner: how professionals think in action*, 1983. New York: Basics Books.

110. Smith, M., Donald Schön: learning, reflection and change, *The encyclopedia of informal education*, 2001.

111. Freshwater, D., Crosscurrents: against cultural narration in nursing. *Journal of Advanced Nursing*, 2000, **32**: pp. 481–485.

112. Freshwater, D., Reflective practice: the state of the art, in D. Freshwater, B. Taylor & G. Sherwood, eds., *International textbook of reflective practice in nursing*, 2008, pp. 2–18.

113. Harris, M., Scaffolding reflective journal writing – negotiating power, play and position. *Nurse Education Today*, 2008, **28**: pp. 314–326.

114. Van Aswegen, E., Action learning through journal writing. *Nursing Update*, 2002. **26**: pp. 52–54.

115. Andriessen, D. *Value, Valuation and Valorisation*, 2005. www.openinnovatie.nl/downloads/Value_Valuation_and_Valorisation.pdf. Accessed 11 November 2008.

116. Peberdy, A., Enquiring and reporting, in J. Katz, A. Peberdy & J. Douglas, eds., *Promoting health: knowledge and practice*, 2000. London: Open University Press: pp. 310–325.

Index

Practical Public Health Nutrition, first edition. Roger Hughes and Barrie M. Margetts. Published 2011 by
Blackwell Publishing Ltd. © 2011 Roger Hughes and Barrie M. Margetts.